Pioneer Programs in Palliative Care:

Nine Case Studies

Robert Wood Johnson Foundation

Milbank Memorial Fund

© 2000 Milbank Memorial Fund

Milbank Memorial Fund
645 Madison Avenue
New York, NY 10022

Printed in the United States of America.

ISBN 1-887748-39-3

TABLE OF CONTENTS

In this report clinicians at nine hospitals describe how they and their colleagues established formal programs of palliative care. Clinicians and managers at each of these institutions negotiated innovative clinical and institutional arrangements and made effective use of the reimbursement policies of public and private payers. Each of these programs of palliative care is a product of the organizational culture of the institution in which it operates.

The nine stories also have common themes. Christine K. Cassel, Professor and Chair of the Henry L. Schwartz Department of Geriatrics and Adult Development at Mount Sinai School of Medicine, who helped to initiate and lead the process that produced this report, describes lessons from the short history of these programs in her introduction. We share her opinion that the success of this report depends on whether it "encourages clinicians who are starting, or who hope to start, palliative care programs in their own institutions."

The report is one result of an ongoing collaboration between two foundations that have similar missions and complementary operating styles. The Milbank Memorial Fund works with decision makers in the public and private sectors to develop better policy for the care of patients, the health of populations, and the organization, financing, and governance of health services.

The Robert Wood Johnson Foundation (RWJF) has as its mission improving the health and health care of all Americans through funding for demonstration projects, training, educational and communications activities, policy analysis, and research. One of its goals is to improve care at the end of life; to that end, RWJF has funded the Center to Advance Palliative Care at the Mount Sinai School of Medicine in New York. The Center's purpose is to serve hospitals and health systems interested in developing palliative care programs at their institutions.

The authors of the studies are identified on the following page. G. Robert D'Antuono, Deputy Director of the Center to Advance Palliative Care, and Beth Demel and Grace Moon, both health policy analysts in the Henry L. Schwartz Department of Geriatrics and Adult Development, Mount Sinai School of Medicine, assisted in the preparation of these stories and in compiling the data that follows each of them.

Daniel M. Fox
President
Milbank Memorial Fund

Rosemary Gibson
Senior Program Officer
Robert Wood Johnson Foundation

THE AUTHORS

Robert M. Arnold, M.D.
Leo H. Criep Professor of Patient Care
Chief, Section of Medical Ethics and
    Palliative Care
Division of General Internal Medicine
University of Pittsburgh
Pittsburgh, Pennsylvania

F. Amos Bailey, M.D., F.A.C.P.
Medical Director
The Balm of Gilead Center
Cooper Green Hospital
Birmingham, Alabama

J. Andrew Billings, M.D.
Director
Palliative Care Service
Massachusetts General Hospital
Boston, Massachusetts

Patrick J. Coyne, R.N., M.S.
Acting Director for Nursing
Massey Cancer Center
Medical College of Virginia Campus of
    Virginia Commonwealth University
Richmond, Virginia

Kathleen M. Foley, M.D.
Member and Attending Neurologist
Pain and Palliative Care Service
Department of Neurology
Memorial Sloan-Kettering Cancer Center
New York, New York

Lachlan Forrow, M.D.
Director
Palliative Care Programs
Beth Israel Deaconess Medical Center
Boston, Massachusetts

Laurel J. Lyckholm, M.D.
Director
Fellowship Program and Palliative
    Care Education
Medical College of Virginia Campus of
    Virginia Commonwealth University
Richmond, Virginia

Diane E. Meier, M.D.
Director
The Lilian and Benjamin Hertzberg
    Palliative Care Institute
Mount Sinai School of Medicine
New York, New York

Jane Morris, R.N., M.S.
Clinical Director
The Lilian and Benjamin Hertzberg
    Palliative Care Institute
Mount Sinai School of Medicine
New York, New York

R. Sean Morrison, M.D.
Research Director
The Lilian and Benjamin Hertzberg
    Palliative Care Institute
Mount Sinai School of Medicine
New York, New York

Richard Payne, M.D.
Chief and Attending Neurologist
Pain and Palliative Care Service
Department of Neurology
Memorial Sloan-Kettering Cancer Center
New York, New York

Thomas J. Smith, M.D.
Medical Director
Palliative Care Program
Medical College of Virginia Campus of
    Virginia Commonwealth University
Richmond, Virginia

Charles F. von Gunten, M.D., Ph.D., F.A.C.P.
Currently: Medical Director, Center for
    Palliative Studies, San Diego Hospice
Associate Clinical Professor, School of
    Medicine, University of California,
    San Diego
Formerly: Medical Director
Palliative Care and Home Hospice Program
Northwestern Memorial Hospital
Northwestern University Medical School
Chicago, Illinois

Declan Walsh, M.Sc., F.A.C.P., F.R.C.P.
    (Edin) (1,2,3)
Director
Harry R. Horvitz Center for
    Palliative Medicine
The Cleveland Clinic Foundation
Cleveland, Ohio

These case studies are stories written by leaders, clinicians who became innovators when they saw the need for palliative care at their hospitals and devoted themselves to creating programs to meet that need. Committed to helping patients live and die without unnecessary suffering, these leaders sought to provide comprehensive care based on respect for patients' goals, preferences, and choices.

Whether they were senior or junior faculty members, all the leaders overcame significant barriers to the development of palliative care within their hospitals. They found varied routes to success, reflecting diverse institutional cultures and differing levels of financial resources, including institutional support that ranged from small to moderate. These pioneers differ, as well, in clinical philosophies, personal styles, and methods of work. Sometimes their subspecialty or research prompted them to act; others were motivated by clinical work. Their personal experiences are an important part of these stories, and their distinctive voices have been preserved in editing the case studies for publication.

The narratives exemplify the current debate that exists about the definition of "palliative care." Is it end-of-life care? Or is it broad and integrated physical, psychological, social, and spiritual care for patients with serious diseases that may be life-threatening?

Most of the authors of these studies believe they should care for patients with advanced, incurable illnesses when aggressive treatment of pain and other symptoms may be needed. Several believe that palliation and cure are not mutually exclusive and that palliative care should be practiced during all stages of serious illness, even while aggressive curative treatment continues. The exact point at which a patient's palliative care should begin remains a subject of discussion.

The authors' programs serve different groups of people and employ diverse clinical models appropriate for particular patient populations. Certain authors developed postacute care linked with hospice and home care. Others created palliative care units or consultation services within their hospitals or have combined both models to provide a continuum of care throughout serious illnesses.

As the charts of financial information show, there is considerable variation in the financing of hospital-based palliative care programs and in institutions' methods of collecting and reporting data. Programs may be supported almost entirely by their clinical revenue or may rely heavily on philanthropy and foundation grants. The charts do not represent all financial activity. They may contain general revenue sources, including research funding, or may break down clinical revenue by payers, depending on a program's ability to report data in a given format.

There is no consensus about how to measure the quality of palliative care. But essential characteristics of hospital-based programs do emerge.

1. Palliative care programs should be constructed around an interdisciplinary team, including at least a doctor, nurse, social worker, pharmacist, and chaplain.

2. Patients, families, and physicians should discuss goals and preferences and should plan the care together.

3. Palliative care should reach patients throughout the hospital, should encourage collaboration across clinical and administrative boundaries, and should foster respect for patients' and families' wishes.

4. Palliative care programs should provide bereavement services for families and staff members.

The impetus for commissioning these case studies was the growing national concern about care at the end of life. There is evidence that acute care settings, especially tertiary teaching hospitals where many barriers impede palliative care, may need the most improvement. At present, palliative care is not formally established as a specialty. Medical culture often equates death with failure. Dedicated revenue streams within institutions are not yet available, and traditional sources of research support, like NIH grants, are few. Nevertheless, patients and their families are overwhelmingly appreciative when a skilled and sensitive interdisciplinary palliative care team offers comfort and dignity to people facing their last days.

Through study or advocacy, a number of projects are now seeking to make end-of-life care more widely available. Possible policy changes include improving the financing of end-of-life care; developing a medical specialty, with board certification, in palliative care; and increasing the quantity and quality of medical education and training in the field.

These pioneers have developed creative ways to surmount obstacles and effect change, and they provide practical advice for other practitioners. This report will be successful if it encourages clinicians who are starting, or who hope to start, palliative care programs in their own institutions. Although these stories are refreshingly diverse, several common threads run through them, like the systemic problems of financial limits and institutional inflexibility. Perhaps the most memorable similarities among the stories, however, are the human qualities— compassion, hard work and, as one author writes, "persistence, persistence, persistence."

Christine K. Cassel

The Balm of Gilead Center
Cooper Green Hospital

F. Amos Bailey

Executive Summary

The Balm of Gilead is a comprehensive program for end-of-life care supported in large part through funding from the Initiative for Excellence in End-of-Life Care of the Robert Wood Johnson Foundation. Cooper Green Hospital, the Jefferson County Department of Health, and the Care Team Network at the University of Alabama at Birmingham (UAB) are partners in the program. We have also established partnerships with local foundations, colleges and universities, religious institutions, civic groups, and professional groups in order to meet the goals of direct service to Balm of Gilead patients and families and education of, consultation with, and outreach to the broader community.

To relieve the suffering of terminally ill patients and their families, the Balm of Gilead Center has created a team of staff, family members, and community volunteers dedicated to providing high quality end-of-life care. This holistic approach emphasizes comfort and pain-free living. Our care incorporates medical, emotional, and social services as well as spiritual care. By supplementing our inpatient services with our hospice services, we can follow the care of our patients effectively.

Gilead has two principal objectives. The first is to integrate existing acute care and end-of-life care throughout Jefferson County. The second is to improve the quality of end-of-life care by developing integrated systems that identify patients who need help earlier in the acute care process; build and coordinate the religious and community resources needed for comprehensive outpatient and inpatient palliative care; and incorporate palliative care into the larger health care system.

The Balm of Gilead Center provides inpatient palliative care for medically underserved people with terminal illnesses who do not have a place to live or do not have support services at home. This 10-bed dedicated unit is located on the fourth floor of Cooper Green Hospital. Each room is furnished and decorated in home-like fashion by a local church or community group.

For those who need home hospice care, the Balm of Gilead Center provides teams of physicians, nurses, clergy, and volunteers who are dedicated to helping families care for their loved ones at the end of life. Through the hospice program of Jefferson County's Department of Health, home-based services are extended to all people regardless of their ability to pay.

Inspiration and Motivation

The Balm of Gilead Center is a community of caring. It addresses the end-of-life needs of people dying in the "safety-net" public health system of the largest county in Alabama. They are relatively young people of color who have little money. At each stage of illness and in each setting of treatment, they and their families receive a continuum of services through the Balm of Gilead Center, including pre-hospice support, inpatient palliative care, home hospice services, and volunteer aid.

My desire to develop palliative care services within the public health system is rooted in my desire for overall high-quality care for the medically underserved. After completing a fellowship in oncology at the University of Alabama at Birmingham, I joined a private practice in the Appalachians as an oncologist and general internist. I later became the medical director of a hospice serving low-income patients in isolated mountain communities. I also began making house calls for homebound patients; a practice I continue today.

In 1994, I was recruited from my private practice for underserved persons in the mountains to a public-health practice for underserved persons in urban Birmingham with the Jefferson Health System and Cooper Green Hospital. I discovered that the percentage of public-health patients in Birmingham who were receiving palliative and hospice care at life's end mirrored the percentage of similar "safety-net" patient populations across America; it was close to

zero. I set out to collect data to substantiate the need for palliative and end-of-life care, and the feasibility of providing it, for these patients.

I developed and administered a three-month survey of inpatients at Cooper Green Hospital, identifying 18 terminally ill medical-surgical patients who needed palliative care. In addition, I found that on any given day from four to seven patients who had been hospitalized for more than seven days could have been discharged if they had had palliative care. However, there were few palliative care services in Jefferson County for people with no home or family or for people whose families were too old, too ill, or too drained by life's other demands to provide consistent care. Such patients, whom treatment could not cure, often awaited death on busy medical units.

The county's home hospice program had eliminated the financial barrier to palliative care by offering its services regardless of insurance status or ability to pay. Thus the county public health system had provided an end-of-life "safety net" for uninsured people whose ages disqualified them from the government insurance reserved for the very young and the very old through Medicaid and Medicare. However, the daily census of the county hospice hovered around seven. Since the average age of home hospice patients was 58, the underuse of the county hospice may have resulted from the preference of aging "safety-net" patients for the private hospice care accessible through Medicare. My hospital survey had shown that inadequate home support was contributing to low hospice use by safety-net patients. I also saw the need to educate physicians and patients about palliative care within the traditional medical delivery system. Under my leadership as the new medical director of the county hospice, its daily census increased from seven to 20; later it rose as high as 35. During this time, I became the first physician in Alabama to be certified by the American Board of Hospice and Palliative Medicine.

I presented the findings of my study to Dr. Max Michael, the CEO and medical director of Cooper Green Hospital. He was highly receptive to my proposal of an inpatient palliative care unit and of hospital-wide adoption of pain assessment and control measures.

Dr. Carole Samuelson, the health officer of the Jefferson County Department of Health, which sponsors the public home-hospice program, was equally receptive. Under my leadership as its medical director, the county hospice had not only seen its daily census increase dramatically but also had become licensed and accredited.

Dr. Michael and Dr. Samuelson saw that if the hospital and the health department collaborated on their clinical and administrative leadership and shared a medical director, their institutions would provide complementary care for the terminally ill. They could envisage a comprehensive program for suffering people within the public health system, a program that would provide compassionate and continuous care through all phases and all treatment settings.

The institutions sealed their collaboration by sending a joint team to the Institute for Healthcare Improvement (IHI) series on palliative and end-of-life care to begin building a team and a cohesive program. Through IHI, the hospital and the department began collaborating with colleagues in end-of-life care across the United States. These colleagues have since provided valuable advice on the inevitable clinical and programmatic challenges that followed. The sense of shared mission with IHI's other safety-net participant, Wishard Health Services of Indianapolis, Indiana, continues to be helpful.

The hospital and hospice began to use their ties with the greater Birmingham community. Collaborators and supporters committed themselves to this innovative effort: to provide excellent end-of-life care for medically underserved people and to spread information about palliative care to the broader community. The two institutions' time and expertise were buttressed by a community-based work group, which helped with program design, grant writing, and local fund-raising to create a "community of caring" at the end of life. The zeal and camaraderie that infused the initial work group and the wide support it enjoys continue to be crucial to the program's success. Before this, the sponsoring institutions had never mobilized and sustained participation in a program by a broad cross-section of the community. That participation is invaluable.

The work group also developed support and collaboration beyond the county government. Generous awards from national and local foundations provided vital financial backing and credibility within the institutions and the community. When the Robert Wood Johnson Foundation awarded the program a three-year grant through its Initiative for Excellence in End-of-Life Care, the combination of funds with external validation infused all participants with energy and confidence. Local foundations, corporations, and religious institutions responded positively to requests that followed. We have established contracts to provide hospice care within local nursing homes and inpatient palliative care for hospices across the county.

Palliative Care Unit

The Palliative Care Unit of the Balm of Gilead Center opened on November 3, 1998. It is a 10-bed dedicated unit within Cooper Green Hospital. Each room is furnished and decorated in home-like fashion by a local church or community group. Inpatient care teams of medical and nursing students who want to serve and learn before assuming a clinical role with patients and their families provide additional support.

Patients admitted to the Palliative Care Unit receive a comprehensive evaluation of their needs by the Center's palliative care specialist and by its medical director. We immediately initiate and carefully monitor palliative care to alleviate pain and to control other symptoms. The palliative care specialist fills a pivotal role by assuring consistency in the continual patient assessments and clinical responses of unit nurses, rotating house staff, and ancillary services. The indispensable contribution of a nurse practitioner to the daily functioning of a palliative care unit had been confirmed for the medical director during his observations as a visiting scholar at Northwestern University.

The medical director provides clinical leadership through daily rounds, 24-hour consultation, and interdisciplinary meetings for review and planning. Serving in his absence is the medical director of the hospice of the University of Alabama at Birmingham (UAB), a close collaborator. This colleague, another Alabama physician who is board-certified in hospice and palliative medicine, is a fellow of the Project on Death in America and has served the Gilead Center since its inception as its consulting psychiatrist and as a member of its Steering Committee. Physicians in training from UAB's Department of Medicine assist the attending physicians and receive their initial exposure to palliative medicine.

To meet social, emotional, and spiritual needs, a multidisciplinary team of physicians, nurses, patient care technicians, clergy, social workers, and volunteers coordinates comfort care. The team spirit of the Balm of Gilead staff, students, and volunteers has been crucial to the Center's daily work and to community support. This "can-do" spirit energizes the team and conveys to the patients and public the compelling nature of the Gilead mission. A social services program helps patients and families obtain a full range of support services across the continuum of care. Through the CareSharing Initiative in cooperation with the UAB Care Team Network, all of the Balm of Gilead Care Team volunteers have been trained in end-of-life care.

The entire interdisciplinary team coordinates holistic comfort care, addressing the four major areas of suffering associated with the end of life, in biweekly meetings where the team reviews the physical, social, emotional, and spiritual needs of each patient and family. Members of the team are highly motivated by their shared mission and by a group ethic that values each member's contribution and each patient's life. Physicians, nurses, patient care technicians, clergy, social workers, administrators, housekeeping staff, students and volunteers, the volunteer coordinator, and rotating home-hospice staff all come together to deal with the multiple challenges faced by dying patients and their personal and professional caregivers. Intensive preparatory training in end-of-life care and two team-building retreats before the unit opened enhanced staff morale and commitment.

The Balm of Gilead Center also reaches out and educates medical providers, patients, students, and the general public. By the end of 1999, the Palliative Medicine Comfort-Confidence Survey had been administered to more than 100 medical residents, interns, and students to assess their knowledge of palliative care. In addition, four third-year residents, eight interns, and eight medical students have attended each monthly in-service session on pain control, during which they received analgesic dosage cards. Since July 1999, the house staff at Cooper Green, consisting of about 20 medical residents and interns a month, have rotated through the

Balm of Gilead. With the assistance of Cooper Green's education department, we have provided continuing education to the Gilead staff on end-of-life care, grief, and bereavement. Balm of Gilead Center staff—F. Amos Bailey, M.D.; John Shuster, M.D.; Carol Padgett, Ph.D.; and Edwina Taylor, R.N.— have conducted monthly in-service training sessions on palliative care at the Jefferson County Nursing Home and have made 15 presentations at the UAB Hospice and during palliative care grand rounds.

The Balm of Gilead Center has provided information to other institutions interested in establishing their own palliative care programs. Representatives from a number of hospitals in Alabama as well as from Wishard Health Services of Indianapolis have visited the unit.

 Home-based Hospice

For those who have adequate family support and choose to die at home, the Balm of Gilead Center provides physicians, nurses, clergy, and volunteer care teams who are dedicated to helping families care for loved ones at the end of life. Through the hospice program of the Jefferson County Department of Health, we extend home-based services to all people regardless of their ability to pay.

During the coordination of home care and care on the inpatient unit, the family or other caregivers receive training in hospice care, end-of-life issues, and bereavement. The hospice staff can also ease the workload on the family. Home health aides help with activities of daily living, such as bathing, eating, or changing linen. Counseling by social workers is available for the patient and family. Chaplains provide spiritual attention and remain available to the bereaved family for up to one year after a patient's death.

From 1998 to 1999, the average daily census of patients in home-based hospice has increased from 22 to 28 patients (a 27 percent increase). Factors contributing to the increase include (1) the efforts by Gilead to identify more patients who need palliative care; (2) the removal of barriers to care through collaborations with volunteers, religious institutions, and social workers; and (3) the enhancement of continuity of care for home-based hospice and the establishment of the complementary inpatient unit.

At the end of life, there is often little continuity of care. Continuity between hospice services in the home and palliative services in the hospital is a hallmark of the Balm of Gilead in all treatment settings. Hospice nurses and chaplains are familiar faces on the inpatient unit, where they stay in close touch with home-based patients who have been hospitalized briefly for symptom control, for a transitional stay between residential placements, or, occasionally, for their final days when family members need support. After a hospice patient dies, the home-based nurse is called to the unit to comfort the family with her familiar presence. Community Care Teams offer practical, emotional, and spiritual support to the patient in the hospital or to the family at home.

The CareSharing and Community Education Initiative

Engaging the wider community is central to Gilead's mission to encourage high quality end-of-life care far beyond its own patients and their families. People from all corners of the community volunteer their personal talents and professional skills to enhance the Balm of Gilead's end-of-life services for county residents with limited resources. Groups of volunteers receive introductory education about end-of-life care based on models used by hospitals, hospices, and care team programs and more advanced education in interaction with patients, their families, and the Gilead staff.

Volunteer care teams of six to ten persons offer practical, emotional, and spiritual support to patients and families in both the hospital and the hospice. Congregational care teams participating in the palliative unit's Adopt-A-Room Program add to the comfort of patients and families. Inpatient care teams of medical and nursing

students who wish to serve and learn before assuming a clinical role with patients and their families provide similar support.

Community Care Teams developed by church, civic, and neighborhood groups form Circles of Care to serve those in the hospice, as well as those who are pre-hospice, during terminal illness and bereavement.

Volunteer professional partners offer specialized skills to patients and families, train clinical staff, and provide valuable aid to the Center's administrative staff. They consult and assist in areas as diverse as research design, data management, legal advocacy, program development, newsletter editing, graphic design, photography, computer training, fund-raising, and referral development. These highly trained persons come to the Balm of Gilead inspired, and leave equipped, to apply their professional skills to end-of-life care.

Undergraduate and graduate students serve and learn at the Balm of Gilead, offering support for patients and families and for Gilead administrative and research projects while simultaneously meeting their own academic and career-preparation goals. One current research study guided by a volunteer academic researcher compares the quality of life perceptions of palliative care inpatients and acute care inpatients who have been matched for severity of illness. A longitudinal study by a doctoral candidate in medical sociology is following patients through their last two years of life to identify factors associated with dying well, as defined by the best current end-of-life practices. A graduate intern in public administration assists the project director in the quality assurance assessment of each program. Student volunteers, in addition to those on the medical student and nursing student care teams, have come from the disciplines of psychology, sociology, human development and family studies, political science, physical therapy, massage therapy, and leadership studies.

This mission to engage the community is guided by Gilead's coordinator of Community Education and CareSharing, who has more than 25 years' experience in clinical psychology as a therapist specializing in the needs of professional and personal caregivers and five years' experience as lay chaplain in the collaborative health ministry of two congregations whose members were primarily elderly. A summary of the personal and professional contributions by people from all walks of life under the CareSharing Initiative follows, detailing the 2,697 hours contributed by 108 volunteers.

Volunteer Care Teams
Trained, supervised volunteers provide practical, emotional, and spiritual support to patients, families, and staff throughout all phases of illness, beginning before the

hospice phase and continuing through bereavement. The support continues within all settings of treatment, including home and inpatient palliative care and post-discharge care in various residential settings.

From November 1998 through September 1999:

- Eight community-based volunteer teams totaling 68 members contributed 835 hours to Gilead patients and families.

- Five church teams from four denominations contributed 373 hours to four families served by the Gilead home-hospice program and to each successive family occupying a church-sponsored room on the Gilead Palliative Care Unit.

- One neighborhood organization team contributed 289 hours to two pre-hospice families and to one hospice family.

- Two teams of first- and second-year medical students contributed 173 hours to patients and families served by the Gilead Palliative Care Unit.

Professional Partners
From November 1998 through September 1999, 20 professionals from fields such as mental health, academic research, pastoral care, music, photography, computer consultation, data management, massage therapy, cosmetology, and barbering volunteered a total of 559 hours during

Gilead's first year—286 in direct patient service and 273 in staff consultation and program assistance. The estimated value of these professional services was approximately $32,000.

Undergraduate Service Learners
From November 1998 through September 1999, 18 undergraduates, who were preparing for careers in various pre-health disciplines at local colleges and universities, contributed 458 hours visiting Balm of Gilead patients and assisting with Gilead research projects and public presentations.

Community Volunteer Visitors
From November 1998 through September 1999, two hospital volunteers choosing service on the Balm of Gilead Palliative Care Unit contributed 10 additional hours of visiting and sitting with patients.

 Dissemination of Best Practices in End-of-Life Care

. . . .

The integration of palliative care into the larger health care system is transforming palliative care in medical settings through consultation, education, and advocacy.

Throughout Cooper Green Hospital, the Balm of Gilead Center provided the leadership and expertise to institute a routine procedure for addressing pain as a fifth vital sign (along with blood pressure, respiration, temperature, and heart rate). The Center developed a visual-analogue scale on which patients regularly indicate the level of their pain, a computerized protocol for staff response to pain, and a monitoring system to ensure prompt response and for adequate pain control. Gilead also developed analgesic dosage cards that show which amount of various drugs correspond to one another. The successful hospital-wide institution of the fifth vital sign project increased staff understanding of palliative care and helped generate the good will and support that has made the new palliative care program welcome throughout the hospital.

Referrals to the consult service provided by Gilead's medical director and its palliative care specialist have increased the frequency of the dissemination of palliative processes throughout Cooper Green. Consultations focusing on alternatives to current and future treatment also provide a natural forum in which to educate medical and nursing colleagues about palliative care methods and about decision making concerning ethical issues. The impact of hospital-wide dissemination of palliative care information is reflected in the dramatic number of terminally ill hospital patients whom physicians referred to the Palliative Care Unit for end-of-life care during its first 12 months—230 patients in all. Physicians' receptivity and referrals can be attributed in part to the staff structure and referral patterns of a public hospital served by one group of salaried physicians. Physicians see patients by rotation, and their referrals to specialty care are not blocked by financial barriers associated with patient "ownership."

Initial steps have been taken to introduce advance directives for health care (ADHC) into the hospital and its clinics. Advance directives are employed on the Gilead unit and in its home hospice. They are a valuable tool used with hospice and hospital patients and families to understand treatment plans and agree upon their goals. The Balm of Gilead developed an interview script for staff members to use when speaking with patients and families. The script is sensitive to the cultural and methodological barriers that may have contributed to the low use of ADHCs by safety-net patients. Interviews using the script have resulted in a much higher rate of acceptance of these documents than previously reported. Implementation of the advance-directive initiative is being delayed, pending review of existing hospital policy that prohibits employees from serving as witnesses for patients' legal documents. An additional barrier to implementation is the forbiddingly long and complex Alabama ADHC itself. In order to complete it, patients need time-consuming help from staff members, but that

help may invalidate the document. A statewide coalition, including the Balm of Gilead, is considering advocating that the legislature adopt the shorter, simpler "Five Wishes" advance directive that is being used successfully in Florida and other states.

Effective practices in bereavement care flow from the Gilead Center into the surrounding community in several ways. The CareSharing Initiative is introducing the practices to more than 50 Community Care Team members and more than 20 volunteers at the Center. In the first three months of this initiative, volunteers on the inpatient unit alone received 360 hours of education about manifestations of grief and its management. Dissemination throughout the hospital has begun with the development of a hospital-wide employee bereavement program.

For this program, Cooper Green's Human Resources Department provides Gilead with the names of employees who have recently experienced the death of a family member. The Human Resources Department also has formalized the existing "grapevine" reporting of family deaths by supervisors. The Balm of Gilead Center immediately mails a condolence letter offering personal and program support to the employee; the letter is signed by the Center's leaders (the medical director, project director, palliative care specialist, charge nurse, and CareSharing coordinator). The first phase of the program has been well received by the hospital's administration and employees.

The Balm of Gilead is now developing a county-wide bereavement program for families served by the entire network of safety-net institutions and clinics. This project will assess population-specific needs in nine domains of life after the death of a family member; identify and coordinate existing intervention options; refer families to community resources; research the outcomes; and advocate affordable, accessible, and population-appropriate services. We have obtained a grant to start staffing the program, beginning with families of Balm of Gilead patients. We are seeking additional grant money for county-wide replication of the pilot program.

The Balm of Gilead staff participates in the palliative care training of medical students and physicians at the University of Alabama at Birmingham. During a regular seminar on pain control, staff distributes analgesic dosage cards monthly to general medicine rotation groups of 20 UAB residents, interns, and medical students. Gilead's medical director leads daily sessions on palliative care while he supervises the rotating medical training groups that learn and serve at the Center. The medical residents in each new rotation group are assessed with the Palliative Medicine Comfort-Confidence Survey. Their responses inform instruction and provide data for longitudinal evaluation of palliative care training. Balm of Gilead staff members have made presentations about the entire spectrum of end-of-life care during UAB's palliative care grand rounds and to wider academic medical audiences at UAB's medicine grand rounds. Gilead staff have designed and introduced the first palliative care curriculum into the UAB School of Medicine. We are developing a UAB–Balm of Gilead Palliative Care Fellowship to ensure the continuing availability of physicians who will sustain Jefferson County's palliative care efforts.

Gilead also disseminates the best practices of end-of-life care to the broader health-care delivery network. The first goal for dissemination beyond Cooper Green Hospital was to develop a contract to provide home hospice services for terminally ill residents of the 250-bed Jefferson County Nursing Home. Both the administration and the nursing staff of the nursing home had serious reservations about the relationship. The administration was wary about sharing costs, reimbursement, clinical responsibility, and clinical documentation with Gilead. The nursing staff resisted palliative care, preferring to transfer patients to a hospital as death approached. Nurses were particularly reluctant to administer analgesics.

The Balm of Gilead program responded to these reservations with friendly persistence, establishing mutually beneficial collaboration as much as possible, regardless of contractual arrangements. Over a number of months, we addressed administrative concerns by clarifying Medicare's hospice regulations and procedures and by building relationships of mutual regard and trust. The medical director began to introduce palliative care to the entire nursing home staff in monthly in-service training sessions, which are continuing. Gilead's palliative care specialist and a home hospice nurse conducted a series of nurse-to-nurse sessions on each shift to provide a forum for frank, collegial discussion of concerns and preconceptions about end-of-life care. These educational efforts provided facts and reassurance and did a great deal to implement the eventual contractual relationship. Soon the hospice census at the Jefferson County Nursing Home was equal to the inpatient palliative care census at the Gilead Center, raising the number of patients in the county's safety-net system who were receiving palliative care at the end of life to about 50 percent of terminally ill patients. We are using this successful process to start collaborations with other nursing homes. The development of contractual relationships to provide palliative care at local nursing homes, especially at the Jefferson County Nursing Home, is an example of the evolution of Gilead's goals as the program learns more about patients' needs.

In response to other emerging, unanticipated realities, Gilead's Palliative Care Unit is trying to supplement its palliative care beds with hospice beds. Patients whose medical condition is appropriate for hospice care but who lack a primary caregiver have encountered barriers to discharge. AIDS patients, whom nursing homes in Alabama have not accepted and whose families often decline to provide care, typically remain on Gilead's palliative care unit without benefit of Medicare hospice coverage to defray the cost. Insured patients whose diagnosis-related group (DRG) coverage has been exhausted during treatment in the referring hospital have encountered barriers to inpatient palliation. When asked what might have been done differently in planning the Gilead program, its medical director quickly answers, "We would have applied for a Certificate of Need for hospice beds on Day One if we had understood the economic realities of hospice and palliative care coverage."

The Balm of Gilead Center has assumed a statewide leadership role in end-of-life issues by participating in the creation of Alabamians for Better Care at Life's End (ABCLE). The coalition will disseminate enlightened understanding about life's final stage and information about the best practices in end-of-life care throughout the state. The Center hosted the organizational

and planning retreat of the group and
continues to formulate and advocate
responsible policies and regulations
concerning end-of-life issues. With the
assistance of funds granted to ABCLE, the
Gilead plans to start a Visiting Rural Scholars
Program, based upon that at Northwestern
University, in which interdisciplinary teams
from each county in Alabama will spend one
week in basic palliative care training at the
Balm of Gilead Center.

I.   Institutional Information

Cooper Green Hospital: The Balm of Gilead Center

Medical Director: F. Amos Bailey, MD, FACP

Date of Initiation: November 1998

Institutional Setting: Urban

Type of Institution: Community Safety-Net Hospital

Number of beds: 319 (10 are located on The Balm of Gilead Unit)

Number of other hospitals within a 20-mile radius: 15

Proximity to other palliative care programs: Another facility is located 250 miles to the south

II. Program Characteristics

   A.   Program Staff

      1.   3 Physicians: The medical director and two other physicians

      2.   Palliative Care Inpatient Unit

         Clinical Staff: palliative care specialist; charge nurse; medical clerk; social worker; 3 LPNs; 4 patient care technicians; 2 unit aides

         Non-Clinical Staff: project administrator; Community CareSharing coordinator; chaplain

         The palliative care specialist, project administrator, and community care sharing coordinator are funded through grants. Other positions are paid through salary.

      3.   Home Hospice

         Clinical Staff: 4 hospice nurses; social worker; registered dietitian; home health aide

         Non-Clinical Staff: administrator; 5 chaplains

         All hospice positions are paid by salary.

      4.   Research Team

         There is no dedicated research staff. However, researchers from local colleges and universities assist staff in studies on various areas of end-of-life care.

      5.   Administrative Staff

         The project administrator's position is funded through a grant from the Robert Wood Johnson Foundation. There is no other dedicated administrative staff.

   B.   The main component of our program is a 10-bed inpatient Palliative Care Unit.

C. Other ancillary programs include:

bereavement support, volunteer services, and caregiver/family support

D. Options for patients after their hospital stay include:

home health care, home hospice care, boarding home with home hospice services, and
nursing home placement with home hospice services.

E. Patient Population:

1. The Balm of Gilead Center had 230 admissions from November 1998 to
September 1999.

2. The average number of admissions per month is 21 (20.9).

3. Diagnoses of patients follow:

DIAGNOSIS	NUMBER	PERCENTAGE (%)
Various forms of cancer	122	53.04
HIV-related illnesses	27	11.74
Cardiovascular diseases	17	7.40
Renal failure	9	3.91
Alzheimer's / Dementia	7	3.04
Pneumonia	7	3.04
Other	41	17.83
Total	230	100.00%

4. Patients by ethnicity:

ETHNICITY	NUMBER	PERCENTAGE (%)
Black	162	70.4
White	62	27.0
Hispanic	3	1.3
Other	3	1.3
Total	230	100.00%

5. Patients by sex:

SEX	NUMBER	PERCENTAGE (%)
Male	136	59.1
Female	94	40.9
Total	230	100.00%

6. Patients by sources of reimbursement:

SOURCE OF REIMBURSEMENT	NUMBER	PERCENTAGE (%)
Medicare	82	35.65
Contracts with local hospices	61	26.52
Medicaid	18	7.83
PMSSI (Possible Medicaid Supplemental Security Income)	13	5.65
Other	17	7.39
Indigent	39	16.96
Total	230	100.00%

F. Budget Information:

THE BALM OF GILEAD CENTER PROGRAM DEVELOPMENT CONSOLIDATED LINE ITEM BUDGET

GRANT PERIOD: OCTOBER 1, 1998—SEPTEMBER 1, 2001

	YR 01	YR 02	YR 03	TOTAL	ROBERT WOOD JOHNSON FOUNDATION 39% OF TOTAL FUNDING	OTHER FUNDING* 61% OF TOTAL FUNDING
I. Personnel	$323,001	$330,816	$341,794	$995,612	$373,905	$621,707
II. Other Direct Costs						
A. Office Operations	8,500	8,700	8,600	25,800	0	25,800
B. Communications	5,000	2,000	2,000	9,000	7,000	2,000
C. Meetings	4,000	9,000	4,000	17,000	0	17,000
D. Travel	6,930	4,650	4,650	16,230	16,230	0
Subtotal	24,430	24,350	19,250	68,030	23,230	44,800
III. Indirect Costs	7,826	6,344	5,688	19,857	19,857	0
IV. Equipment	5,000	0	0	5,000	0	5,000
V. Contractual	20,000	20,000	20,000	60,000	30,000	30,000
Total	$380,257	$381,510	$386,733	$1,148,499	$446,992	$701,507

*Other funders are Cooper Green Hospital, the Jefferson County Department of Health, and five local foundations.

SOURCE OF FUNDING	AMOUNT	PERCENT
Local foundations (In-kind support for the Balm of Gilead)	$175,000	15.2%
Cooper Green Hospital and the Jefferson County Department of Health (Matching funds for the Balm of Gilead)	$526,507	45.8%
The Robert Wood Johnson Foundation (Initiative for Excellence in End-of-Life Care)	$446,992	39.0%

G. Home Hospice Component: (Birmingham Area Hospice)

The Birmingham Area Hospice served 145 patients in fiscal year ending September 1999. Data during that fiscal year follow:

- **REVENUE SOURCES BY PERCENTAGES**

1997	1998	1999
42% Medicare	38% Medicare	39% Medicare
32% Medicaid	24% Medicaid	28% Medicaid
20% Non-insured	29% Non-insured	30% Non-insured
5% VA (Veterans Administration)	6% VA	1% VA
1% Third party	3% Third party	1% Third party

- **ADMISSIONS**

Number of admissions: 134 Total Patient Days: 7712

Average length of stay (ALOS): 71 days (51 days, NHO avg.; 58 days, AL avg.)

"Average length of stay includes only the deceased and discharged patients (NHO)"

ALL PATIENTS SERVED DURING FY1999 (145)

Average daily census (ADC): 28

Total number of visits to patients by discipline:	5,164
Nurses	2,882
Social workers	607
Home health aides	1,026
Clergy	553
Volunteers	47
Number of days by level of care:	11,130
Routine	10,744
Continuous care	0
Respite care	12
General inpatient care	374

- **PATIENT SUMMARY**
  - 54% were male and 46% female. 20% of the males and 36% of the females were over 66 years old. 41% of the males and 36% of the females were between 51 and 65 years old.
  - The average age was 56. The youngest patient was 15. The oldest was 96.

- 70.4% of the patients were black. 26% were white.
- Of the 145 patients served during FY1999, there were 111 deaths. 22 died on the Balm of Gilead unit (20%); 74 (68%) in the home; 2 (2%) at Ketona, 3 revoked, 9 discharged, and 1 transferred.
- **MAJOR DISEASE CATEGORIES PER 111 DEATHS OR DISCHARGE:**

Lung cancer	18%
Breast cancer	12%
AIDS	12%
Colon cancer	6%
Prostate cancer	4%

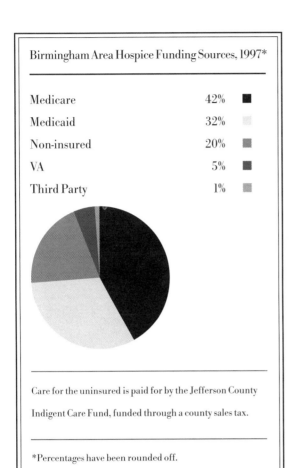

Birmingham Area Hospice Funding Sources, 1997*

Medicare	42%	■
Medicaid	32%	□
Non-insured	20%	■
VA	5%	■
Third Party	1%	■

Care for the uninsured is paid for by the Jefferson County Indigent Care Fund, funded through a county sales tax.

*Percentages have been rounded off.

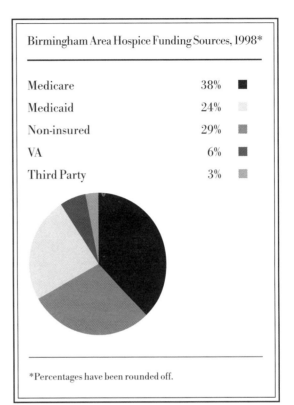

Birmingham Area Hospice Funding Sources, 1998*

Medicare	38%	■
Medicaid	24%	□
Non-insured	29%	■
VA	6%	■
Third Party	3%	■

*Percentages have been rounded off.

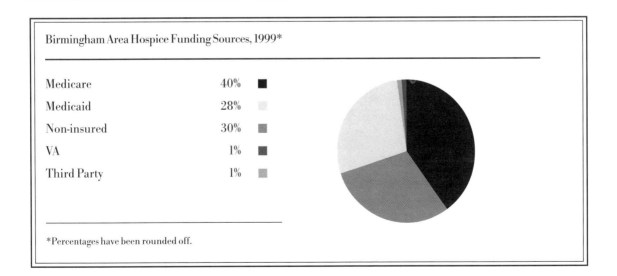

Birmingham Area Hospice Funding Sources, 1999*

Medicare	40%	■
Medicaid	28%	□
Non-insured	30%	■
VA	1%	■
Third Party	1%	■

*Percentages have been rounded off.

Palliative Care Programs
Beth Israel Deaconess Medical Center/ CareGroup

Lachlan Forrow

Executive Summary

Beth Israel Hospital and Deaconess Hospital, which merged in October 1996 to form Beth Israel Deaconess Medical Center (BIDMC), had each been strongly committed to improving the care of patients near the end of life. The 1995 results of the SUPPORT study, for which Beth Israel Hospital had served as a site, had demonstrated serious inadequacies in the care of patients with life-threatening illnesses. Survey results using Picker Institute instruments documented additional shortcomings in important dimensions of "patient-centered" care.

At the time of the merger, many pieces of a comprehensive palliative care program already existed, including a 15-bed inpatient hospice unit established at Deaconess Hospital in early 1996, an affiliated outpatient hospice system, and the region's largest pain center. Senior leadership enthusiastically encouraged initial efforts to build an overall palliative care program from these components, and the clinical staff welcomed them. But progress during the next two years was limited. Substantial organizational stresses related to the merger, major turnovers in institutional leadership, and a rapidly worsening financial environment—including unprecedented staff layoffs—required that top priority be given to programs that could directly improve the organization's fiscal stability. At the same

time, the integration of BIDMC and several other institutions into CareGroup, a unified regional health care delivery system, brought new opportunities to plan and implement more effective palliative care across the continuum of inpatient and outpatient services.

With crucial and timely support through the Faculty Scholars Program of the Project on Death in America, BIDMC and CareGroup leaders made a renewed two-year commitment in 1999 to support the development of a comprehensive palliative care program. Most important was the provision of operating budget support for a full-time nurse and for .4 FTE (full-time equivalent) physician time to staff a new Palliative Care Consultation Service. Systems for careful documentation and evaluation of the impact of this Service, and of the entire palliative care program, upon patient-centered measures of clinical quality and upon finances were established. The continuation or expansion of palliative care beyond 2001 will depend on the results of those evaluations.

General Organizational Background and Current Context

Brief History of BIDMC and CareGroup
The Boston Jewish Community founded Beth Israel Hospital in 1916 to meet the

needs of a growing immigrant population. Deaconess Hospital, founded in 1896, had as its mission the support of Methodist deaconesses in caring for the city's residents. These independent, Harvard-affiliated academic medical centers were located within two blocks of each other in Boston's Longwood Medical Area. After they merged in October 1996, Beth Israel Deaconess Medical Center integrated all clinical and administrative operations into one organization, with a single board of trustees, a single chair or director of each clinical and financial or administrative department, and a single operating budget. BIDMC included 625 inpatient beds and 1,145 staff physicians serving more than half a million patients annually in and around Boston, with strong links to urban community health centers serving inner-city minority communities and to suburban medical practices.

At the same time that Beth Israel and Deaconess merged to form Beth Israel Deaconess Medical Center, BIDMC joined with Mount Auburn Hospital, New England Baptist Hospital, and several suburban Boston hospitals to form CareGroup. CareGroup was designed as a network that would bring important benefits to participating institutions and their affiliated physician practices through collaborative negotiation of contracts with insurers and suppliers and through streamlined

information systems, referral systems, and other medical and practice management services. With BIDMC as its principal tertiary/quaternary academic hub, the CareGroup network included more than 14,000 employees, more than 1,800 medical staff members, and more than 1,500 acute and subacute beds. The network would serve the community through more than 60,000 annual discharges, more than 400,000 annual outpatient visits, and approximately 280,000 home care visits.

The three years following the BIDMC merger and the simultaneous formation of CareGroup brought enormous organizational change, even turmoil. There were challenges in integrating previously independent organizations, and external changes in health care financing created tremendous pressures. Financially, BIDMC encountered major operating losses after the merger, including an operating deficit of over $40 million in FY1999 alone, leading to unprecedented staff layoffs. The initial displacement of numerous senior administrative and clinical leaders, when many positions were consolidated, was followed by a second period of major leadership turnover. Since mid-1997, almost all top management positions within BIDMC have changed hands, within the administration and in the leadership of clinical departments, including medicine, surgery, psychiatry, nursing, and social work.

CareGroup has experienced analogous changes during the second and third years of its existence. Just two years after it began in 1996, CareGroup was restructured from a network of semi-autonomous institutions to a fully integrated corporation with a single operating budget and corresponding bottom line. After an operating surplus of nearly $28 million in 1997, its first fiscal year, CareGroup's financial position worsened considerably, with an overall operating loss of approximately $100 million out of a total budget of approximately $1.2 billion for FY1999. Like BIDMC, CareGroup saw major transitions in its senior leadership during this period. Twelve of 16 senior management positions changed hands during 1998–99.

Amid these organizational upheavals, it was difficult to develop any new clinical initiatives, like an enhanced palliative care program, that required the consistent support of leaders or the allocation of new financial resources. Nonetheless, we made important progress that built upon the programmatic strengths and organizational values of Beth Israel and Deaconess Hospitals. The growing documentation of inadequate end-of-life care, other U.S. institutions' success in improving its quality, and the increasing recognition that current care near the end of life was likely to be contributing to the medical center's financial difficulties all contributed to further progress.

Pre-Merger Beth Israel and Deaconess Leadership in End-of-Life Care
Both Beth Israel Hospital and Deaconess Hospital had been pioneers in palliative care before their 1996 merger. As far back as 1927, Palmer Memorial Hospital was established under the auspices of the New England Deaconess Association, dedicated to the care and treatment of cancer patients and other "incurables." In the early 1990s, Deaconess Hospital was one of the first sites for Decisions Near the End of Life, a program sponsored by the Kellogg Foundation and the Educational Development Center (EDC). Among the fruits of this program were a heightened institutional interest in end-of-life care and a published manuscript showing that regular ethics rounds in the Deaconess Surgical Intensive Care Unit led to fewer prolonged, ultimately futile, ICU stays, and improved both the quality of care and the hospital's finances (Holloran et al., 1995). In April 1996 Deaconess Hospital established a 15-bed inpatient hospice unit on campus, as described below.

Beth Israel Hospital (BIH) brought its own record of leadership to the merger as creator in 1972 of the first patient's bill of rights, as a pioneer in DNR policies and procedures during the mid-1970s (Rabkin et al., 1976), as the location for Frederick Wiseman's widely acclaimed six-hour 1990 documentary "Near Death," and as one of five national sites for the landmark SUPPORT study. Suzanne Gordon's 1997 book *Life Support: Three Nurses on the Front Lines* reinforced Beth Israel's reputation for excellent care of patients with life-threatening illnesses by recounting the work of the BIH nursing staff in delivering personalized care to seriously and terminally ill patients on inpatient floors, in oncology, and in home settings.

Documentation of Need for Improvements in Patient-Centered End-of-Life Care
....

Organizational Pride Confronts Empirical Data: The SUPPORT Study
In 1988, Beth Israel Hospital had been pleased to be chosen as one of five U.S. sites for the five-year Study to Understand Prognoses and Preferences for Outcomes and Risks of Treatments (SUPPORT), sponsored by the Robert Wood Johnson Foundation. Proud of its reputation for leadership in patient-centered care, most staff at the hospital expected the SUPPORT study to confirm Beth Israel's reputation for excellent care near the end of life. The November 1995 report of the results provided a stiff antidote to that organizational confidence. All five participating institutions showed severe shortcomings in end-of-life care, and

Beth Israel was no better than the others in any important way. The shortcomings, documented exhaustively in various SUPPORT publications, included findings that:

- 38 percent of enrolled patients who died spent at least 10 days in an intensive care unit;
- for 50 percent of conscious patients who died in the hospital, family members reported moderate to severe pain at least half the time; and
- only 47 percent of physicians knew when their patients preferred to avoid CPR.

Beth Israel did not solve any of these problems during an intervention phase in which SUPPORT staff, including specially hired and trained clinical nurses, worked to improve communication and decision-making by providing timely and reliable prognoses to attending physicians; to elicit and document patient and family preferences and understanding of prognoses and treatment; to help plan pain management; and to convene family meetings and other discussions to facilitate care planning. Virtually all interventions involved individual patients, one at a time. The hospital did not undertake any institution-wide interventions, because of the need to follow a control group of patients within each institution.

While Beth Israel's staff accepted the overall validity of the SUPPORT study, they did not believe that the failure of the intervention phase meant that hospital-based efforts to improve end-of-life care were doomed. They concluded that efforts to transform such care would require institution-wide changes involving methods that the SUPPORT study's design had not permitted. Exactly what those changes should be, however, was far less clear.

Limitations in the Institutional Impact of the SUPPORT Results

Several features of the SUPPORT study's design and findings made them hard to act upon. As disturbing as the aggregate results were, BIH staff members who were directly involved in the intervention phase of the trial (myself included) had difficulty identifying, even in retrospect, specific cases involving clinical care contrary to the wishes or preferences of a patient or a patient's family or involving prolonged and avoidable suffering. For example, the stereotypical individual "horror story" of a SUPPORT patient, which was presumed to be common from the aggregate results, concerned a patient whose physician was ignorant of the patient's desire to avoid CPR, who spent a prolonged period in the ICU in the days leading up to death, and who often had moderate to severe pain during the terminal phase of the illness. But the

nursing and medical staff who participated in the intervention phase believed that most prolonged ICU stays that culminated in death stemmed largely from ambivalence on the part of patients and families about accepting the terminal nature of the illness; it took substantial time for patients, families, and clinical staff to reach the consensus that a shift to comfort-oriented care was appropriate (Hiltunen et al., 1999).

In addition, the aggregate, institution-wide nature of the SUPPORT study's results did not indicate that specific individuals, clinical departments, or service units had particular responsibilities or opportunities for improving care. This contrasted with other data-driven quality-improvement efforts, such as those from the Picker Institute, in which patients' reports about shortcomings were directly linked to the clinical units where care had been delivered, and in which nurse managers and medical and administrative staff on those units who could do better in the future were identified and held accountable. Finally, the fact that no site in the SUPPORT study had done any better than BIH left uncertainty about the extent to which the shortcomings could be corrected within a single institution. The problems suggested a need for broader social change in the way patients, families, and clinical staff approached life-threatening illnesses in general and the prospect of death in particular.

Nonetheless, in the wake of the SUPPORT study, I had encouraging initial discussions with BIH leaders about developing and implementing an institution-wide effort to improve end-of-life care in late 1995 and early 1996. Hospital administration put this effort on hold before formal activities could begin, however, as plans for the merger with Deaconess Hospital became serious in the first half of 1996. The discretionary funds for a new initiative, which were tentatively identified in late 1995, were no longer considered available by mid-1996, primarily because transitional costs of the merger were anticipated.

The Picker Institute and Broader Institutional Quality Issues
Dr. Thomas Delbanco, chief of BIH's Division of General Medicine and Primary Care, founded the Picker Institute in 1987. Started as the Picker/Commonwealth Program for Patient Centered Care, the organization was launched through support from Harvey Picker, whose company, Picker X-Ray, invented the CAT scan, and from the Commonwealth Fund, a private New York-based philanthropic institution. Picker began by investigating discrepancies between routine assessments of patient satisfaction, which are generally high in the healthcare industry, and reported patient experiences that often suggested

fundamental flaws in the quality of care. For example, although half of all patients in the SUPPORT study reported pain, and moderate to severe pain near the end of life was frequently reported by patients or their families, only 15 percent of patients with pain expressed dissatisfaction with its control, perhaps reflecting a reluctance to criticize care and a fatalism about the inevitability of pain, which is unnecessary in light of modern pain management techniques (Desbiens et al., 1996).

Building from focus groups of patients that identified core "dimensions" of "patient-centered care," Picker developed a standardized method for surveying patients after their discharge from U.S. hospitals, in which patients were asked to *describe*, rather than *rate*, the care they received. The Picker Institute, which was incorporated as a nonprofit affiliate of Beth Israel Hospital in 1994, currently provides patient-survey services to more than 400 health care organizations. Twenty-five dimensions of care comprised of 138 questions from Picker Institute adult and pediatric questionnaires have been approved as clinical measures for the ORYX initiative of the Joint Commission on Accreditation of Healthcare Organizations (JCAHO). The Veterans Administration has adopted Picker surveys as its national standard, with more than 250,000 veterans surveyed since 1994.

Although Beth Israel had begun using early Picker instruments to assess quality of hospital care by 1989, organization-wide attention to Picker "scores" was heightened dramatically in 1997. Through the Massachusetts Health Quality Partnership, a coalition of insurers and business and professional groups, 58 of Massachusetts's 76 acute care hospitals agreed to provide a random sample of recently discharged patients for Picker surveys. Results from surveys early in 1997 would be confidential, with each institution receiving its own scores together with blinded results from other participating hospitals. The 1998 scores would be distributed in the same way at first, but unblinded scores would be made public later and widely disseminated, allowing open comparisons among institutions.

The BIDMC–Picker results in early 1997 attracted immediate and intense attention throughout the organization. They showed that BIDMC's results were no better than the Massachusetts-wide average on multiple dimensions of care. Within selected dimensions of care, such as "continuity and transition" from the inpatient setting to subsequent outpatient care, BIDMC's results were worse than the statewide average. These results challenged the organization's self-image as a national leader in compassionate, patient-centered care at least as powerfully as any of the SUPPORT

results. For example, despite Beth Israel's proud pioneering role in creating the first hospital patient's bill of rights, the Picker survey showed that BIDMC was ranked only average among participating Massachusetts hospitals regarding "respect for patients' values, preferences, and expressed needs," with 16 percent of patients reporting problems of this kind.

Perhaps more important, the Picker results seemed to have clear and direct implications for quality improvement activities, in striking contrast to the uncertain implications of the SUPPORT results. In this regard, four fundamental differences between the Picker and SUPPORT results stand out. First, although both studies were "comparative," the Picker findings demonstrated distinct differences among institutions, strongly suggesting that change within an institution could lead to better results in the future. Second, the Picker findings for each institution were linked to the specific clinical units where patients had received care; different BIDMC units had different scores. This provided accountability so that nurse managers and others could improve their units' performance. Third, the Picker surveys would be repeated at regular intervals, so that improvements in performance—or the lack of them—by individual units and by the medical center as a whole would become evident over time. Finally, the knowledge that 1998 Picker scores would be publicly released provided a powerful incentive for everyone from the leaders of the Board of Trustees on down to achieve as much positive change as possible in a short period of time, before a large institution-by-institution table was published in the *Boston Globe*.

1996–1998: Forward Steps and New Hurdles

. . . .

Creation of the Palliative Care Center (1996)
While Beth Israel Hospital was grappling with the implications of the SUPPORT study in late 1995, nearby Deaconess Hospital was planning for improved end-of-life care of its own. The chief landmark in the development of today's BIDMC palliative care program was Deaconess's creation of its 15-bed inpatient Palliative Care Center in April 1996. In part because the Decisions Near the End of Life Program had stimulated institutional awareness of end-of-life care, hospital leaders wanted to explore ways to meet patient and family needs more effectively and less expensively than in the hospital's acute care beds. In this exploration, Dr. R. Armour Forse, director of the Surgical Intensive Care Unit, played a crucial role. He had learned the importance of a formal palliative program during his training at Canada's Royal Victoria Hospital, an internationally renowned leader

in the field. Deaconess leaders spent over a year assessing the possibility of contracting with HealthCare Dimensions, a local hospice organization, to organize an inpatient hospice unit in the hospital's Palmer Building.

The average number of deaths per year at Deaconess Hospital at this time was approximately 350. To weigh the need for inpatient palliative care, the hospital conducted two "demand analyses" in early 1995, surveying all Deaconess inpatient units. The data from the assessments were inconsistent. In January 1995, of 225 patients surveyed by non-clinical staff, we identified 35 as having life-limiting disease, only three of whom we identified as being appropriate for admission to a palliative care unit. The following month, other staff, including Dr. Forse and a hospice nurse, surveyed 263 patients, identified 19 of them as being appropriate for admission to a palliative care unit, identified another 60 as patients who would benefit from a palliative care consultation, and identified nine more as needing palliative care at home. The combined data from these two analyses suggested that a 12- to 15-bed inpatient palliative care unit might be justified by the needs of Deaconess inpatients.

A Deaconess Hospital committee charged with evaluating the proposed Palliative Care Center identified the following pros and cons:

"Opportunities"

- Coordinate palliative, clinical, teaching, and research activities
- Provide integrated continuity of care through an interdisciplinary team of healthcare professionals and volunteers
- Increase revenue through rental income from HealthCare Dimensions, the hospice organization
- Decrease variable costs by reducing the length of stay
- Add convenience and other benefits for patients who could stay in a familiar inpatient environment
- Use the expertise of HealthCare Dimensions to provide skilled staff
- Develop a cooperative model between Deaconess and HealthCare Dimensions for family support and bereavement

"Concerns"

- HealthCare Dimensions needs an average daily census of nine patients to break even financially
- Referral mechanisms to promote effective patient flow need to be developed
- Competition for space on the Deaconess campus

Given the discrepancy between the January and February 1995 inpatient surveys, the Deaconess Hospital financial staff needed to anticipate the consequences of changing the care of current inpatients. According to one estimate, a 12- or 13-bed occupancy derived entirely from Deaconess inpatients could "save" 2,792 inpatient days. At a conservative estimate of $150 in variable costs saved per day, the medical center would reduce its costs by $400,000 by transferring inpatients to a more appropriate setting.

In April 1996 Deaconess Hospital and HealthCare Dimensions signed a contract establishing a 15-bed inpatient hospice in the hospital's Palmer Building. In compliance with Medicare hospice regulations, this unit was managed and staffed by HealthCare Dimensions, rather than by Deaconess personnel. HealthCare Dimensions paid annual rent for the space and was able to admit and care for patients qualifying for inpatient hospice services, while avoiding many administrative and financial burdens of creating its own inpatient hospice facility. Deaconess Hospital agreed to provide all routine inpatient services for a base per diem rate, including pharmacy services, meals, housekeeping, and laundry. The hospital also agreed to ensure that adequate facilities were available for flexible visits by families, including overnight stays.

As a result of this contract, Deaconess Hospital now had an on-site hospice unit to which acute care inpatients who were too ill to go home could easily be transferred. From an administrative perspective, patients were "discharged" from Deaconess Hospital to HealthCare Dimensions. Deaconess hoped that these patients and their families would experience a high degree of continuity in care during the transition from acute to palliative care, since the "transfer" actually involved only a change of floor or building on the hospital campus. In addition, patients and families would have the broad benefits of hospice care, including bereavement services for family members. Deaconess also counted on some reduction in the number of prolonged stays that significantly exceeded Medicare DRG reimbursement, while acknowledging that objective evidence that this would ensue would be difficult or impossible to obtain. The financial staff calculated that an average daily census of nine patients would produce enough money to cover the hospital's costs of providing care on the unit.

Since 1996, more than 1,000 patients have received care on the unit, with a mean length of stay of just over 20 days but a median stay of only nine days. Approximately 20 percent of patients have died within three days of admission. The vast majority of patients have died on the unit. A small fraction have been able to return home for their terminal care.

A relatively consistent average daily census of greater than nine patients (recently

11.5 patients) has resulted in an operating surplus for the unit. But the fact that the unit remains the only inpatient facility of its kind in Massachusetts has caused an unexpected, sometimes problematic, pattern of referrals. Up to 75 percent of referrals in some months have come from acute care hospitals, with half or more than half coming from outside of BIDMC. In addition, patients transferred to the PCC from other home hospice organizations have transferred their Medicare hospice benefits to HealthCare Dimensions upon admission. Because Medicare regulations require that a certified hospice provide at least 80 percent of its patient-care days in a home setting, and because a substantial number of the Palliative Care Center's patients receive no home care through HealthCare Dimensions, many inpatient PCC days are not offset by any preceding home hospice days. That has at times required HealthCare Dimensions to refund to Medicare part of the revenues the organization received for inpatient hospice care. In the future, this may be addressed in part through separate contracts with other referring hospice organizations for inpatient PCC hospice care within the referring hospice's Medicare benefit.

One primary financial benefit of the PCC that BIDMC hoped for was the reduction in acute care inpatient stays, beyond DRG reimbursement, for terminally ill patients. No systematic assessment of the extent to which this has actually occurred has yet been undertaken.

Creation of a BIDMC End-of-Life/Palliative Care Working Group (1997)

Dr. Joanne Lynn's presentation at medical grand rounds in January 1997, as part of the BIDMC-*JAMA* "Clinical Crossroads" series, helped spark renewed efforts to address the inadequate care that had been documented by the SUPPORT study. With the support of Dr. Jennifer Daley, co-editor of "Clinical Crossroads," who was at the time also BIDMC vice president and medical director for healthcare quality, a team from BIDMC joined the Institute for Healthcare Improvement (IHI) Breakthrough Series Collaborative on Improving Care Near the End of Life in July 1997. Team members included Dr. Forse, surgical ICU director; Marjorie Wiggins, director of nursing with oversight responsibility for the inpatient hospice; and me, a general internist and director of the medical center's Ethics Support Service. Through individual meetings with nurse managers on every inpatient unit and with other medical, nursing, social work, and pastoral staff, we formed a broad interdisciplinary network of nearly 50 staff members interested in improving end-of-life care, and a Palliative Care Working Group of 12 to 15 people began to meet monthly to plan activities. A smaller group led by Wiggins and me met weekly.

By August 1997, a detailed analysis of existing programs was prepared, identifying these building blocks of a comprehensive BIDMC/CareGroup palliative care program:

1. The 15-bed inpatient Palliative Care Center described above

2. Affiliation with HealthCare Dimensions, the largest outpatient hospice provider in the region, which had become a wholly owned CareGroup subsidiary through consolidation of the institutions affiliated with CareGroup

3. The largest pain management center in the region, including a chronic and cancer pain program, with more than 8,000 patient visits annually

4. A Division of Oncology whose director, Dr. Lowell Schnipper, served as head of the End-of-Life Task Force of the American Society of Clinical Oncology

5. The second-oldest home care program in the region, with more than 350,000 visits annually

6. The BIDMC Patient/Family Learning Center, whose recent focus groups of families of patients who had died at BIDMC led to a new initiative providing hands-on instruction to other families in the technical skills they need to keep their loved ones at home

7. The Center for Alternative Medicine Research, directed by Dr. David Eisenberg, which had documented in two recent studies that approximately 70 percent of BIDMC oncology patients and approximately the same number of HIV patients use alternative therapies for symptomatic or curative goals. (Fairfield et al., 1998).

These resources, however, were not being coordinated. Working Group members agreed that all of the pieces of a comprehensive palliative care program would be in place with the addition of an inpatient Palliative Care Consultation Service. In September 1997, a letter of intent was submitted to the Robert Wood Johnson Foundation requesting support for such a service under the foundation's new program, Promoting Excellence in End-of-Life Care. The Service would come under the auspices of a proposed BIDMC/CareGroup Center of Excellence in Palliative Care. Dr. Mitchell T. Rabkin, CEO of CareGroup, pledged $225,000 in new institutional funds to supplement the requested $450,000 in RWJ support. Unfortunately, BIDMC's proposal to RWJ was not successful, nor was my January 1998 application to the Faculty Scholars Program of the Soros Foundation's Project on Death in America.

The process of preparing the unsuccessful RWJ and Soros/PDIA applications nonetheless had the vital benefit of bringing Working Group members together to formulate an overall mission and vision statement and program goals for BIDMC/CareGroup palliative care, with input and subsequent endorsement from both BIDMC and CareGroup leaders. The statement and goals (Table 1) have remained essentially unchanged since their adoption in 1997.

Program Goals:

1. To provide prompt, interdisciplinary, and comprehensive palliative care consultation services that meet the needs of BIDMC patients and families who confront life-threatening or life-limiting illness, and that enhance the clinical excellence of physicians, nurses, and others who are responsible for their care.

2. To provide educational programs that create and sustain palliative care knowledge and skills of the highest order throughout the BIDMC and CareGroup communities.

3. To create systematic programs throughout CareGroup that will transform the quality of care that patients and families receive near the end of life, sharing ideas and achievements with the communities we serve and with others working in this field, locally, nationally, and internationally.

Table 1. Excellence in End-of-Life/Palliative Care: The BIDMC/CareGroup Vision

Mission: To ensure the delivery of life-affirming palliative care services of the highest quality to all BIDMC/CareGroup patients and families who need them.

Life-affirming palliative care:

1. is always anchored in realistic and carefully-considered *goals and values of the patient*

2. includes prompt and effective *treatment of physical and emotional symptoms* and enhancement of *functional status*

3. provides support for patients and families struggling to find or create *affirmative meaning* in the last stages of life

4. ensures that patients and families experience *continuity in care* during transitions across settings of care

5. helps families prepare for and manage the financial and other *burdens* of life-threatening illness

6. includes *bereavement services* for family members after the patient's death

7. ensures that all services are provided in sites and with personnel that are as *cost-effective* as possible, with *adequate reimbursement* to ensure high quality today and improved quality in the future

8. offers *effective training* of the health care professionals and volunteers who will provide tomorrow's end-of-life/palliative care, helping them to develop the *skills* they will need and to sustain their professional energy for, and fulfillment in, this work

9. provides *public education* about death and dying that helps create a social context that facilitates effective end-of-life/palliative care

10. is ultimately *evaluated* by the *reported experiences* and overall *satisfaction* of our patients and their families

4. To conduct research that strengthens and expands the knowledge needed to improve palliative care.

The IHI Breakthrough Series (1997–1998): Limited Immediate Results

Tangible results from BIDMC's involvement in the 1997–98 IHI Breakthrough Series Collaborative were disappointing. One of the first goals chosen, given the disturbing SUPPORT findings of inadequate pain control, was to improve the documentation and results of pain management on selected inpatient medical and surgical units where most hospital deaths occurred. However, leading physicians and nurses in the ICUs, where half of all inpatient deaths take place, did not perceive serious shortcomings in pain control on their units, where most gravely ill patients were heavily sedated. A subsequent Harvard-wide study of patient and family satisfaction with ICU care, which included four ICUs at BIDMC, revealed such a high level of satisfaction in the baseline phase that it was difficult to design any quality improvement strategies to achieve better outcomes. This confirmed for ICU directors at BIDMC that patients and families preferred prolonged ICU care in the face of otherwise terminal illness, and that the ICU problems that the SUPPORT study documented would have to be reduced by addressing patient and family expectations

for care, and attitudes toward death, long before patients reached an ICU.

Initial steps to encourage nursing staff on one of the general medical units, with nearly 100 deaths annually, to record pain as a fifth vital sign by documenting the frequency of pain levels greater than five on a 10-point scale found fewer than 5 percent of patients with levels that high, a percentage so low that the staff did not consider a major unit-wide change in pain assessment to be worthwhile. At about the same time, Picker survey results showed that BIDMC's results for "physical comfort" were considerably better than most Massachusetts hospitals. Higher institutional priority was given to improving clinical care in other areas, where BIDMC's Picker scores were average or below.

More progress was made in efforts to improve staff education. Nearly 200 BIDMC clinicians, primarily nurses, participated in day long educational programs related to palliative care, including pain management, during 1997–98. A much larger number took part in shorter events, including enthusiastically received medical and surgical grand rounds presentations that described the mission and goals of BIDMC/CareGroup palliative care activities. In addition, we started weekly, hourlong palliative care rounds on two inpatient units, to which nursing staff and, occasionally, medical staff would bring a current case of a patient whose palliative care needs were not being adequately addressed. Staff took extensive notes during the sessions on a laptop computer, creating a log of nearly 100 cases. These sessions were useful for documenting in detail the need for new inpatient palliative care. They gradually built up staff members' interest in evolving palliative care activities and helped us understand in very concrete terms the problems that the Service would need to address. This approach also helped prevent us from duplicating services. In many cases, important patient or family needs that were not being met could be met through existing services, by the pain service or by referral to home hospice or to the Palliative Care Center.

Initial Commitment to Operating Budget Support for Expanded Palliative Care Services
Post-merger difficulties in integrating Beth Israel and Deaconess administrative and clinical activities continued to consume much of the time and energy of Palliative Care Working Group members who might otherwise have been available for additional program development. An additional serious barrier was the lack of any BIDMC staff position specifically funded to support further program development, although the IHI Collaborative had explained from the start that reliable progress would require at least one .5 FTE position.

Following the unsuccessful applications to RWJ and Soros/PDIA for extramural support, and in light of the documented gap between palliative care needs and services, the Palliative Care Working Group appealed to the BIDMC administration for operating budget support, explaining that there was little purpose in the group's continuing its work without it. BIDMC's senior vice president and chief operating officer, Robert Norton, immediately agreed to support the inclusion of approximately $125,000 in funds for the FY1999 budget, which would support .4 FTE in physician time (half of it already provided in FY1998 for leadership of the BIDMC Ethics Support Service), .4 FTE of a clinical nurse specialist to assist with a Palliative Care Consultation Service, and .4 FTE of administrative support. His decision was clearly based on his earlier central role in discussions about creating the Palliative Care Center. These had convinced him that expanded palliative care could improve both the quality of care and BIDMC's bottom line. Although the PCC had proven itself financially viable through direct hospice revenues, many of the bed days were filled by patients referred by other Boston-area hospitals, as already noted, and considerably more financial advantages seemed likely if more BIDMC inpatients were referred to the unit in a timely way.

Impact of Staff Changes and Increasing Institutional Financial Difficulties

Shortly after the FY1999 budget lines were approved in principle, BIDMC's overall financial projections for the fiscal year were revised significantly. BIDMC implemented an institution-wide "austerity budget," freezing new staff positions, erasing budget lines for new educational activities, and reducing hours for some nurses and other staff. After her hours were reduced by eight hours a week, the clinical nurse specialist who had spearheaded the highly successful palliative care education programs left for a full-time position at another hospital; that largely educational staff position was later discontinued. In late 1998 and early 1999, four champions of the palliative care initiative left to take senior positions at other institutions, including CEO Bob Norton, Surgical ICU Director Dr. Armour Forse, Director of Nursing Marjorie Wiggins, and Vice President and Medical Director for Healthcare Quality Dr. Jennifer Daley. Dr. Jim Reinertsen replaced the retiring Dr. Mitchell Rabkin as CEO of CareGroup, and many other senior leadership changes in both BIDMC and CareGroup followed.

During the mid-1999 development of the FY2000 BIDMC budget, the challenge of reducing an anticipated FY1999 operating deficit by nearly $40 million led to the first layoffs that Beth Israel personnel had experienced in decades, including the reduction of Social Work Department staff on inpatient services by nearly 50 percent.

1999: Some Breakthroughs

Reframing of Palliative Care Issues in the Context of Financial Problems

Given the medical center's financial plight, it became clear that requests for support of any new initiative, such as enhanced end-of-life care, would need to be justified not only in terms of improved quality but also—if not primarily—in terms of their net effect on the institution's fiscal stability. Meetings with BIDMC financial staff led to a rapid agreement to assess the financial implications of current end-of-life care.

The results were summarized in a March 1999 memorandum to senior BIDMC/CareGroup leaders:

1. *For Patients Dying in Acute Care Beds.* During FY1998, the 776 adult patients who died in acute care beds accounted for nearly $36 million in hospital charges during their final admission alone. Those "terminal hospitalizations" generated more than $20 million in "actual" (variable) costs but only $14.8 million in actual revenues, for a total contribution to the operating deficit of nearly $5.5 million for FY1998.

2. *For Patients Dying under Hospice Care.*
Financial results of end-of-life care
through the hospice services of
HealthCare Dimensions were
dramatically different, despite a year of
its own institutional turmoil, including
three executive directors in rapid
succession. With 810 admissions and
19,347 patient-care days, HealthCare
Dimensions incurred $3,600,000 in
expenses and received $3,066,000 in
patient care revenues. With the addition
of $350,000 in charitable
contributions, the HealthCare
Dimensions operating deficit for the
terminal care of 810 patients was
$184,000. Given the improved
organizational stability and
infrastructure resulting from its
successful retention of its latest
executive director, HealthCare
Dimensions predicted a balanced
operating budget for FY2000.

3. *Dangers (including Financial!) of
Focusing on Financial Outcomes.* The
memo to BIDMC/CareGroup leaders
stressed that "Efforts to approach this
primarily as a 'cost-reducing' endeavor
are likely to fail or even backfire." It
acknowledged that many of the 776
patients who died in BIDMC's acute
care beds had undoubtedly received
technologically intensive, expensive life-
prolonging efforts beyond what they or
their families would have wanted if
other choices, like world-class palliative
care, had been available. But the memo
warned that an effort to encourage any
of the 776 patients and families to
consider palliative care that hinted that
the hospital wanted to save money
would further erode already-fragile
trust, would likely make decision-
making "even more difficult," and could
easily result in still longer ICU and other
acute care inpatient stays.

4. *Proposed Solutions.* The memo offered
two recommendations to address the
problem:

a. BIDMC should make a major
institutional commitment to creating a
comprehensive, first-class Palliative
Care Program that will be attractive to
clinicians, patients, and families. This
program would build from the existing
inpatient hospice unit in the Palmer
Building and the outpatient services of
HealthCare Dimensions, the hospice
provider owned by CareGroup.
Support for a full-fledged BIDMC
Palliative Care Consultation Service,
already well advanced in planning,
would soon be very important.

b. BIDMC should provide support, in
connection with CareGroup's Center
for Quality and Value, for developing

methods for tracking the quality, use patterns, and costs of care near the end of life. For assessments of quality, the Picker Institute had recently received two years of funding from RWJ to develop and validate patient- and family-centered instruments dealing with end-of-life care. The analysis that led to the successful establishment of the Palliative Care Center at Deaconess Hospital in 1996 remains valid: use a system-wide approach for cost analyses. For example, hospice or other palliative care services might be reimbursed below cost for some patients, but reimbursement might have been even lower had they remained on acute care floors.

Senior BIDMC and CareGroup leaders expressed strong support in principle for the memo's conclusions that care near the end of life is one of the few areas where the elusive goal of better quality at lower cost is in fact attainable and that the BIDMC/CareGroup could become a regional and national leader in this field. Initially, however, the pressing problem of BIDMC's projected $40 million deficit for FY1999, which demanded reduced direct expenditures and increased direct revenues, meant that the administration could not immediately translate support in principle

into operating budget support for enhanced palliative care.

Crucial New Support from the Soros/PDIA Faculty Scholars Program

In reapplying to the Soros/PDIA Faculty Scholars Program, I included a letter of support from Dr. Reinertsen, CEO of CareGroup, that summarized the analysis and conclusions of the memo described above. I also included a letter from Joyce Clifford, BIDMC senior vice president of nursing, stating that if I were chosen then BIDMC would guarantee its original FY1999 commitment of $125,000 per year in operating support through FY2000 and FY2001. With my selection in April 1999 as a PDIA Faculty Scholar for 1999–2001, the combined funds from BIDMC and PDIA allowed the creation for FY2000 and FY2001 of a new full-time position for a clinical nurse specialist to serve as the hub of a Palliative Care Consultation Service, a budget line supporting .4 FTE physician time on the Service, and slightly expanded administrative assistance. During the budgeting process, it became clear that, without the prior written commitment from Joyce Clifford, who had since retired, in the Soros/PDIA application, approval of the palliative care budgets for FY2000 and FY2001 would have been extremely unlikely. No institutional financial commitment existed beyond the end of

FY2001. Continuation of any operating support for palliative care services would depend on a clear demonstration of their quality and cost implications.

In addition to its crucial role in ensuring funding for the first two years of an inpatient Palliative Care Consultation Service, my selection as a 1999–2001 PDIA Faculty Scholar supplied other major boosts to the palliative care efforts. Palliative Care Working Group members were reenergized. Internal organizational credibility was increased by the implicit Soros/PDIA endorsement. In the summer of 1999, the Working Group sought and obtained a small grant from the Kenneth B. Schwartz Center to develop reliable systems for providing information about bereavement to family members of BIDMC inpatients who had died and for contacting them afterward to offer referrals for further services. In the fall, Iris Cohen, a member of the Social Work Department, successfully applied for the new Soros/PDIA Social Work Leadership Development Award, receiving two years of support for training social workers and physicians to work with patients and families in establishing patient-centered care plans for patients with life-threatening illnesses.

BIDMC Palliative Care Center Featured in PBS Broadcast
Unexpected and invaluable new support for BIDMC palliative care arrived when the weekly PBS broadcast *Religion and Ethics Newsweekly* chose the Palliative Care Center for a June 1999 story on how end-of-life care could be life-affirming for patients, families, and clinical staff. We showed copies of the seven-minute video, which followed three PCC patients, to senior BIDMC and CareGroup leaders and trustees. They saw more vividly than in any memo that excellent end-of-life care could inspire internal and external organizational pride. Two subsequent issues of the medical center's monthly publication, *Our News,* featured the Palliative Care Working Group's efforts. We regularly incorporated the video in many other presentations and conferences.

2000–2001: Implementation and Evaluation of the Palliative Care Program

With the hiring of a full-time nurse practitioner supported by attending physician staff, the long-sought BIDMC Palliative Care Consultation Service was launched in February 2000. Its planning had built upon knowledge gained from palliative consultation services established elsewhere, including those at Massachusetts General Hospital, Mount Sinai Hospital and Beth Israel Medical Center in New York, and the University of Pittsburgh, and upon additional guidance from the network of Faculty Scholars in the Project on Death in

America. We developed four components of a comprehensive approach to palliative care.

1. *Early Identification of Inpatients with Potential Palliative Care Needs.* Beginning with a pilot program on one medical unit in November 1999, the unit's nurse manager reviewed all admissions with medical house staff and nursing case managers each day, asking them to identify any patients for whom death within the next 12 months would not be a "surprise." This approach, used successfully by PDIA Faculty Scholar Dr. Neil Wenger on several inpatient units at UCLA, identified patients who would be the primary targets of proactive outreach efforts by the consultation service and who would also form a cohort to be tracked for evaluation.

2. *Outreach by the Palliative Care Consultation Service.* In addition to responding to any spontaneous requests for palliative care consultations, the Service's nurse practitioner and attending physician would seek out nursing staff, house staff, and attending physicians and ask whether there were any palliative care needs that could be addressed through informal or formal consultation. They would place a brochure describing the range of

BIDMC palliative care services— including formal consultation, hospice and home care services, and bereavement programs—in the medical chart. (Dr. Wenger found at UCLA that the placing of even a single page, designed to spark thinking about overall goals of care, led to a dramatic increase in chart documentation of discussions of care goals, advance directives, and DNR status.) Adapting a simple format used by Dr. Diane Meier and her colleagues at Mount Sinai, the Service would document in its own records any formal or informal recommendations made to clinical staff, as well as a subjective sense of the extent to which staff implemented those recommendations. Specific issues arising from any of these interactions with each unit's clinical staff then become the basis for regular in-service training of nursing staff and for discussions with house staff during rounds by attending physicians.

3. *Tracking Use and Cost.* With support from Dr. Risa Burns of the CareGroup Center for Quality and Value, a system was established in November 1999 to track the use, costs, and reimbursements, both prospectively and for the preceding 12 months, for all patients identified as potentially

needing palliative care services. Use included admissions, emergency unit visits, length of stay, medication, laboratory services, and the like. Three months of data collection before the inpatient consults began would provide baseline data for later comparisons. These data, which would be generated automatically through standard medical center information systems, would be linked to additional information about BIDMC/CareGroup hospice and home care use that required allocated time from an administrative assistant and staff in those clinical areas.

Subsequent analyses would attempt to discern whether formal or informal engagement of the Service was related to any changes in use, cost, and reimbursement. For example, favorable trends in referrals to CareGroup's hospice organization, HealthCare Dimensions, could increase the average length of stay on hospice, with financial benefits to HealthCare Dimensions and thus to CareGroup's bottom line, which could in turn be used to justify continued investment in inpatient consultations.

4. *Patient- and Family-Centered Quality Measures.* As the March 1999 memo to BIDMC/CareGroup leaders

emphasized, the most important justification for enhanced palliative care is not financial benefit but improved quality of care. In contrast to the well-established Picker instruments used in evaluating acute hospital care, the lack of a proven, easily used instrument with which to elicit systematic reports from patients and families about their experiences in end-of-life care, with results that can be readily incorporated into quality-improvement activities, continues to be a major gap for all institutions across the United States. Through its close affiliation with the Picker Institute, BIDMC has already begun to serve as the primary hospital site for the pilot phase of the development and testing of a Tool Kit of Instruments to Measure End of Life Care (TIME), sponsored by the Robert Wood Johnson Foundation. This will ultimately include an after-death survey instrument that will examine the patient's overall quality of life; patient and family experience in decision making with health care providers; symptom management; and family-centered reports about the quality of care. Additional instruments will cover bereavement services, the psychological distress of family members, family experiences before and after the patient's death, and spirituality and transcendence. The staff members leading this project at Picker and at Brown University, under Dr. Joan Teno, plan to develop a resource guide and computer software to facilitate use of these tools for evaluation and quality improvement. BIDMC will be deeply involved in these efforts.

 Conclusions

. . . .

The ups and downs of efforts to enhance palliative care at Beth Israel Deaconess Medical Center since 1995 provide several important lessons:

1. Hospital leaders' enthusiastic support for a new program, which began in late 1995 and was often reaffirmed, is inadequate without financial resources.

2. Organizational stresses accompanying a merger can create extremely high barriers to program development, but persistence in promoting the program can ultimately succeed despite frequent major changes in organizational leadership.

3. External support, like that provided to BIDMC through the Faculty Scholars Program of the Project on Death in America, can be crucial not only directly but also by mobilizing internal resources.

4. When institutions face financial difficulty, no new program is likely to succeed unless its potentially favorable financial implications are highlighted. Yet, a primary focus on financial measures of success is extremely dangerous.

5. Although quality assessment in the field of end-of-life palliative care is only in its infancy, in the long run, measurable improvements in quality are likely to provide the strongest justification for continued support of a clinical program.

NUMBER OF PATIENTS ADMITTED TO

INPATIENT HOSPICE UNIT:

1996:	124
1997:	268
1998:	305
1999:	325

GENDER: (AVERAGE 1996–98)

Male:	50.1%
Female:	49.9%

AGE DISTRIBUTION: (1996–98)

18–64:	33%
65–74:	24%
>74:	43%

INSURANCE:

Medicare:	74%
Medicaid:	6%
Commercial:	20%

INCOME/EXPENSES (FY1999):

Figures represent total revenue and expenses for HealthCare Dimensions, and therefore includes both home hospice and inpatient palliative care.

Net Patient Service Revenue:	$3,086,526
Other Operating Revenue:	$ 12,528
Net Fundraising Revenue:	$ 231,140
Total Revenue:	$3,330,194
Total Expenses:	$3,527,572
Total Gain/Loss:	($197,378)

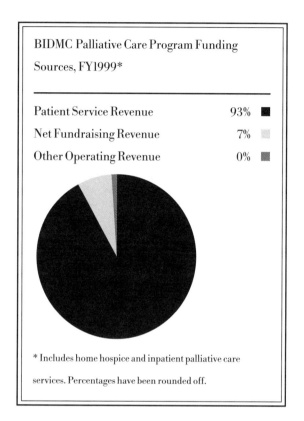

BIDMC Palliative Care Program Funding Sources, FY1999*

Patient Service Revenue	93%	◼
Net Fundraising Revenue	7%	◻
Other Operating Revenue	0%	◼

* Includes home hospice and inpatient palliative care services. Percentages have been rounded off.

Project on Death in America:

July 1, 1999–June 30, 2001 $76,500/year x 2 years

Support for Dr. Lachlan Forrow's work as a 1999–2001 Faculty Scholar, with primary focus on developing BIDMC Palliative Care Programs.

Project on Death in America:

January 1, 2000–December 31, 2001 $30,000/year x 2 years

Support for the work of Iris Cohen, LICSW, in the Social Work Leadership Development Award program, developing interdisciplinary education for medical and social work personnel and assisting the BIDMC Palliative Care Programs.

Kenneth B. Schwartz Center:

October 1, 1999–September 30, 2000 $20,000

Support for development of bereavement activities within BIDMC Palliative Care Program.

REFERENCES

Desbiens, N.A., A.W. Wu, S.K. Broste, et al. 1996. Pain and Satisfaction with Pain Control in Seriously Ill Hospitalized Adults: Findings from the SUPPORT Research Investigations. *Critical Care Medicine*, 24:1953–61.

Fairfield, K., D. Eisenberg, et al. 1998. Patterns of Use, Expenditures, and Perceived Efficacy of Complementary and Alternative Therapies in HIV-Infected Patients. *Archives of Internal Medicine*, 158(20):2257–64.

Hiltunen, E.F., C. Medich, S. Chase, L. Peterson, and L. Forrow. 1999. Family Decision Making for End-of-Life Treatment: The SUPPORT Nurse Narratives. Study to Understand Prognoses and Preferences for Outcomes and Risks of Treatments. *Journal of Clinical Ethics*, 10(2):126–34.

Holloran, S.D., G.W. Starkey, P.A. Burke, et al. 1995. An Educational Intervention in the Surgical Intensive Care Unit to Improve Ethical Decisions. *Surgery*, 118(2):294–8.

Rabkin, M.T., G. Gillerman, and N.R. Rice. 1976. Orders Not to Resuscitate. *New England Journal of Medicine*, 295:364–6.

The Harry R. Horvitz Center for Palliative Medicine, The Cleveland Clinic Foundation

Executive Summary

The Cleveland Clinic is a large multispecialty group practice. The clinic identified the need for a palliative care program, and the program started in 1987. The structure of hospice care as Medicare defines it is inadequate for incurably ill patients. Palliative medicine implies physician expertise in the areas of: communication, decision-making, management of complications, symptom control, care of the dying, and psychosocial care.

Since 1987, the program has established a hospital consultation service, outpatient clinics, acute care inpatient service, hospice/home care service, an acute care palliative medicine inpatient unit, which evolved from our acute care inpatient service, and an inpatient hospice facility. We have introduced a new component approximately every 18 months since the program began. These activities have considerable implications for staffing, the management of change, and the competition for scarce resources within a shrinking health care budget.

For staffing, the program has turned to specialized attending physicians, using a multidisciplinary approach to enhance the role of nursing. The major budgeted areas are the acute care Palliative Medicine unit and the hospice/home care service. To develop an intellectual basis for the practice of palliative medicine, we have made a commitment to systematic research and education. Senior leaders within the Cleveland Clinic Foundation, including the Cancer Center, have consistently supported the program.

The major lessons learned during program development have been: to focus on the quality of patient care; to pursue research and education; to secure institutional commitment to program development; to establish a businesslike approach; to defend the program's budget and personnel during this difficult period in health care; and never to promise anything that you do not deliver.

The Cleveland Clinic Foundation

The Cleveland Clinic Foundation is a private nonprofit group practice founded in 1921. It integrates clinical and hospital care with research and education. There are 850 full-time salaried physicians representing more than 100 specialties and subspecialties. The main hospital has almost 1,000 beds. Last year 1.2 million outpatient visits and 50,000 hospital admissions occurred in the foundation's two main hospitals in Cleveland, Ohio, and Fort Lauderdale, Florida. Through a series of expansions, mergers, and acquisitions, the foundation has grown to include 10 community hospitals in the greater Cleveland area as well as 15 family health centers and a number of other specialized clinics and health care facilities, among them the Harry R. Horvitz Center for Palliative Medicine (Walsh, 1990). For administrative purposes, Palliative Medicine is a subsection of the Department of Medical Oncology within the Cleveland Clinic Taussig Cancer Center, which is located in urban Cleveland. There are no other palliative care programs in greater Cleveland.

The Philosophy of Palliative Care: Hospice or Palliative Medicine?

. . . .

The conviction that the principles and practices of palliative medicine must be incorporated into the acute medical care system have governed our program (Walsh, 1994a). These principles and practices derive from the hospice model but have been modified to fit into mainstream medicine. A major deficiency of U.S. hospice care has been its separation from acute care structurally, administratively, financially, and philosophically. The initial impetus for hospice services was in part a reaction to deficiencies in health care. As a result, nurses and social workers have dominated U.S. hospice care administratively and philosophically, in

contrast to hospice in the United Kingdom, where physician's leadership has been common. Indeed some U.S. hospice programs are antiphysician. Moreover, the structure of Medicare's hospice benefit excludes physicians from many hospice services. These influences have damaged the development of hospice and palliative medicine in the United States. Many hospices have been isolated from the medical community and from the acute care system, with late referrals and a short length of stay a major problem. Palliative medicine in this country is at least a decade behind that in western Europe.

We believe that hospice philosophy needs to be integrated into acute care and into the entire fabric of health care. This is the key difference between the concepts of palliative medicine and hospice. Providing hospice services, as defined by Medicare, is an important part of our program but does not define our philosophy or practice. Being part of the acute health care system, palliative medicine should be delivered in the same fashion as other health care services, judged by the same clinical, administrative, and financial standards, and held to the same level of accountability (Goldstein et al., 1996). We must also compete with other programs for resources, space, and funding. Health care in the United States is changing significantly under internal and external stresses. Program development in any area is fraught with difficulties and complexities, particularly when the field of medical endeavor—palliative medicine—is new. Yet postacute services for chronically ill elderly people will play an expanding role in palliative medicine as the U.S. population ages.

 Mission Statement

The mission of the Palliative Medicine Program is to:

- Provide excellent care for patients with advanced cancer and their families throughout the illness and during the bereavement period.
- Advocate comfort, dignity, and choice for patients.
- Gain international recognition through clinical excellence, comprehensive research, and a commitment to education at all levels.

At the Cleveland Clinic Foundation, Palliative Medicine is an integral part of the Department of Hematology and Medical Oncology. The program provides multiple clinical services on a continuum of medical care, and patients can obtain access to it 24 hours a day, seven days a week. Primary medical care is provided, rather than a consultation model. Due to its multiple revenue streams, the program is financially self-supporting.

Clinical Competencies in Palliative Medicine

The development of palliative medicine is hampered because this discipline is not clearly defined. Based on our experience since 1987, we identify six components of clinical expertise as essential to palliative medicine. These not only define the practice but underpin the education and research needed to advance the field.

Communication
When disease is advanced, communication is often ineffective. The information imparted to patients and families is haphazard and disorganized. Miscommunication often results in pseudoethical problems, concerns about legal implications, and daily frustration due to clinical chaos in complex medical environments. Effective communication within the medical team is essential. Otherwise there is no plan of care. Indecision rapidly reaches patient, family, and nursing staff, with predictable results. In daily practice, better communication within the medical team(s), with the patient, and with the family and caregivers can improve this situation (Miller, Krech, and Walsh, 1991).

Decision-Making
Choices about care during life-limiting, complex diseases depend on effective

communication (Stagno, et al., 2000). Decisions about the direction of care are difficult and dynamic. They require knowledge of the natural history and unpredictability of common illnesses and their complications. Options for care may cover a wide range, including aggressive interventions such as laparotomy, discontinuation of treatment, or sedation of the dying patient.

Management of Complications
Many common complications of advanced disease are predictable (Nelson et al., 2000a). For example, the common problems in advanced cancer can often be identified by the cancer's primary site, allowing a structured approach to its management if intervention is appropriate. Although many complications are everyday occurrences, few hospitals have devoted systematic clinical, educational, or research activity to their management. This stands in stark contrast to the excessive expenditures devoted to developing ineffective cancer therapies. The absence of well-defined and widely accepted protocols for managing such complications, like hypercalcemia, is a noteworthy deficiency of modern cancer care.

Symptom Control
Relief of symptoms in advanced disease is a primary responsibility of palliative medicine

(Walsh, 1997; 2000). When an individual cannot be cured, sophisticated control of symptoms by pharmacologic and nonpharmacologic intervention becomes urgent. Because of the interplay between palliative medicine and acute care, we believe that all modern technologies that relieve symptoms, such as esophageal stents, should be used. Appropriate use of these interventions depends on excellent communication and decision-making. Under "low-tech" care at hospice, patients may inadvertently be denied "high-tech" interventions that relieve suffering.

Care of the Dying
Despite the predictability of many deaths in an acute care setting, death is often a chaotic and depersonalized process with poor communication, ineffective decision-making, and bad symptom control. As a result, many dying persons suffer unnecessarily. The essential responsibility is to decide whether a patient is in fact dying. Once this decision has been made many complexities of end-of-life care resolve themselves because decision makers choose among realistic care options. Palliative medicine offers ways to manage care of the dying while considering the needs of the care team and the family, and focusing upon the patient most of all (Miller and Walsh, 1991; Nelson et al., 2000b).

Psychosocial Care

In addition to the multiple physical symptoms associated with advanced disease, many patients and their loved ones suffer considerable psychosocial distress (Miller and Walsh, 1991). Beyond the common problems of anxiety, depression, insomnia, and the like lie many other stresses like financial difficulties or the disruption of long-term human relationships. Humanitarian values play a central role in medical practice under palliative medicine. We deliberately try to elevate and incorporate humanitarian values and practice good medical care at the same time. The values and the care are not mutually exclusive. A philosophical commitment to psychosocial care means dedicating resources, personnel, and energy to it. Improved communication and decision-making can relieve much psychosocial distress by clarifying people's roles, the care plan, and the predictable problems. Discussing the prognosis, delivering bad news, and maintaining a continuing relationship with the patient and family as the center of care all afford considerable relief to the patient and family and to the staff caring for them.

 ## Program Development

Our program is based on the model developed by Balfour Mount at the Royal Victoria Hospital in Montreal, Canada. We wanted to build a similar program, physically located within the main hospital complex and routinely included in the spectrum of medical services (see Table 1) (Ahmedzai and Walsh, 2000; Tropiano et al., 2000). The major difference between our program and the one at Royal Victoria is that our inpatient unit is an acute care unit while their inpatient unit is more hospice-oriented.

Consultation Service

In the fall of 1987, program development began with a consultation service staffed by an attending physician (me), a nurse clinician, and a part-time social worker. At first, consultations in the hospital were the only clinical services provided. The need for outpatient clinics for follow-up of patients after consultations and discharges were soon obvious.

Outpatient Clinics

The second part of the program, outpatient clinics, provide continuity of care after hospital consults and discharges. Once the clinics started, outpatient consults followed. The clinics are located in the cancer center, alongside traditional oncology clinics. The clinics are solely for palliative medicine and are open five afternoons a week.

Home Hospice Care

Until our own hospice service began, we

Table 1: Palliative Medicine Program History	
1987	Inpatient consult service
1988	Outpatient clinics
	Board of advisors
	Research program
1989	Inpatient service
	Education program
	Physician fellowship
1990	Home hospice care service
	Nursing fellowship
1991	World Health Organization designation
1992	Palliative care scholars program
	Cancer home care service
1994	Harry R. Horvitz Palliative Medicine Center
1995	Hospice expansion
1996	Regional conference on palliative medicine
	Harry R. Horvitz Chair in Palliative Medicine
1997	National conference on palliative medicine
	Professional advisory board
1998	Hospice inpatient unit
1999	Integration with postacute care services

referred discharged patients to local home care and hospice programs where appropriate. But there were problems with the consistency and quality of care in the home and problems of coordination with the hospital. The palliative medicine program was also losing revenue that would have been valuable to program development. In 1990, we decided to begin our own home care and hospice service. The hospice has been linked to the Cleveland Clinic Foundation since then. It serves metropolitan Cleveland and some surrounding counties.

Acute Care Inpatient Unit

The acute care inpatient unit, our program's fourth component, was established in 1994. The average length of stay is 7–10 days. Traditional health insurance and Medicare under the DRG system fund care. Hospice patients are among those admitted for management of medical complications and acute care symptoms. But the unit is not a hospice. We do not admit patients simply because they are dying.

Inpatient Hospice Unit

Following the development of the acute care inpatient unit and the home hospice service, it became clear that we needed beds where hospice patients could stay for longer periods and for respite care. We have contracted with local nursing homes to dedicate beds for our hospice. Our program conducts inservice training for the staff in these units. We also provide case management by nurses and backup by attending physicians.

Thus we have added a major component to the program about every 18 months since palliative medicine services began. This has demanded a significant commitment of energy and resources in order to maintain momentum and let the program develop quickly. Nevertheless, it has taken over a decade to start these services. That time span illustrates the complexity and difficulty of developing new programs and ensuring that they will be effective and fiscally responsible.

 Administrative Structure

· ·

Nursing Case Management
The program began by instituting nursing case management. Every new patient referred to the program was assigned a registered nurse as case manager. The nurse (1) serves as the routine contact for the patient and family; (2) performs triage on patients with complex illnesses during acute care; (3) adjusts medications within defined limits, using protocols similar to those of hospice nurses; (4) participates in outpatient clinic visits and consultations; and (5) acts as liaison with community resources, including home health agencies, nursing homes, and

hospice services. The nurse brings intimate knowledge of the health care system and of the needs of patients and families to bear on each complex, changing case.

Business Plan
We felt it was essential to develop a formal business plan for palliative medicine, on the grounds that a totally new concept in medical care would be judged more stringently than established services (Walsh et al., 1994b). This proved to be correct. The written plan presented to, and approved by, various hospital administrative bodies considerably eased the development process. It was tangible evidence that detailed work and forethought were going into program development. The plan reassured senior administrators that this service was necessary and valuable and that it was being handled in a fiscally responsible manner.

The first business plan was for the establishment of the home hospice of the Cleveland Clinic. Approval by senior administrators allowed us to start one of the first home hospice services in the United States directly owned and managed by a tertiary care medical center. We used the hospice business plan as a model for the later palliative medicine business plan, which incorporated elements of the hospice proposal but covered education, research, and clinical services.

This planning has enabled us to meet

the overall goals of the Cleveland Clinic Foundation. It demonstrated our sense of purpose in establishing and meeting objectives that were tied to schedules. We published the business plan so that similar programs at other institutions could use parts of it in their own proposals. We hoped that a published business plan would also lend legitimacy to program development at other institutions.

Reimbursement and Palliative Medicine
There is a perception that clinical services for palliative care cannot be reimbursed. But if the services are part of the acute medical care system, reimbursement is available for medical consultation, inpatient and outpatient care, and hospice. A consultation or outpatient service alone is not financially viable. In our view, the service must make a commitment to provide primary medical care. Reimbursement from Medicare and other payers is subject to the same vagaries as all other areas of clinical activity today. All

payers want only to cut costs, giving lip service to the quality of care.

Medicare will always be a key reimbursement source for palliative medicine because of the age of the people most likely to need it and because of nationwide demographic trends. The Medicare hospice benefit needs to be restructured. It creates an artificial health care structure for persons with advanced disease, in conflict with its original intent. A structure based on needs should be substituted, in which the hospice benefit is added to existing acute care reimbursement, not substituted for it (Walsh, 1998).

The structure of our program is designed to maximize clinical (Figure 1) and financial integration. Each clinical area can stand alone as an individual service line. Activity in one area, however, automatically supports and increases activity in all others (Figure 2). The revenue stream that activity in each area creates contributes to the program's overall financial health to ensure

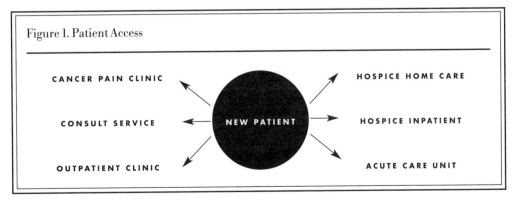

Figure 1. Patient Access

CANCER PAIN CLINIC

CONSULT SERVICE

OUTPATIENT CLINIC

NEW PATIENT

HOSPICE HOME CARE

HOSPICE INPATIENT

ACUTE CARE UNIT

its survival. The multiple revenue streams that home hospice, consultations, and inpatient care generate are all important to any hospital department or system. This is particularly true given that these revenues were largely lost to our hospital system before the development of Palliative Medicine, primarily because patients needing palliative care tended to be sent back into the community, often in adverse circumstances.

Our program's five major areas—consultation, outpatient clinics, home hospice, acute inpatient care, and inpatient hospice—allow rapid, flexible access for the patient and the referring physician (see Figure 1). Services can meet the patient's needs anywhere in the trajectory of an illness. The program responds quickly to emergencies. No matter what the specific problem is, we can always respond, whether with admission to an acute care unit, urgently needed consultations, or assessment of the situation at a patient's home by a nurse. These responses are also important as indirect marketing, creating an image of the program as a dynamic, dedicated part of the acute health care system. It is essential to avoid the perception that palliative care is "fluff."

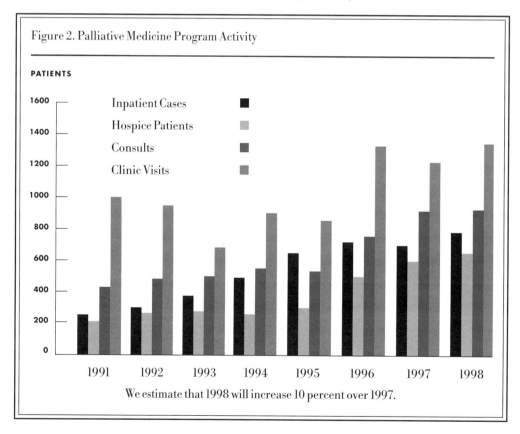

Figure 2. Palliative Medicine Program Activity

PATIENTS

- Inpatient Cases
- Hospice Patients
- Consults
- Clinic Visits

We estimate that 1998 will increase 10 percent over 1997.

Complementary clinical services demonstrate that palliative medicine is comprehensive and integral to the entire health care system. Improved patient satisfaction and increased revenue are important in promoting palliative medicine internally. Externally, they generate community support and philanthropic contributions for still more palliative care services.

Funding
Our business plan showed that palliative medicine produces as much net income as other areas of medical oncology. Patient revenue predominantly funds our program. The Department of Medical Oncology supports our nurse clinicians. Small but significant philanthropic donations continue to support staff education. We have not applied for any grants.

Staff Comments
Medical professionals find palliative medicine rewarding. Asked what aspect of their work offers the most satisfaction, staff members answered:

"...the constantly changing, unpredictable course of the illness and its meaning for the patient and family." —Ruth Powazki, M.S.W.

"...knowing that in some way I've made a difference in a patient's life by not being afraid to try and answer difficult and awkward questions at a very difficult time of their life." —Denise Brady, R.N., nurse clinician

"the ability to promote symptom management for the medically complex patient."—June Olson, R.N., assistant nurse manager

"...a great sense of professional and personal fulfillment in the knowledge that people can trust me enough to help them handle one of the most intense and intimate times of their lives." —Mary Kay Stahley, R.N.

Pamela Tropiano, R.N., B.S.N., nurse manager, has commented, "I have learned to always base my management decision on what is best for the patient."

I myself enjoy the complexity of the medical care, the constant challenges. I admire the bravery of the patients and believe that we have done our best for them and their families even in difficult circumstances.

Staffing

. . . .

Attending Physicians
The program has four full-time attending physicians. All are board-certified in Internal Medicine and Medical Oncology. Two of the

attendings also practice part time in traditional chemotherapy-based Medical Oncology. The attending physicians are allocated annual study time, based on their seniority, as well as an opportunity to attend an annual educational conference.

Nursing Staff

Two nurse clinicians are dedicated to the program. In addition the inpatient unit has a full nursing staff (see Table 2). The home hospice service has all the required disciplines, including the nurses required for Medicare certification. A director who is in charge of the acute care palliative medicine inpatient unit and the home hospice service provides nursing leadership. In addition, she supervises the part-time nurse practitioner and the two nurse clinicians.

Ancillary Programs

Because hospice is Medicare-certified, we provide the full range of bereavement, volunteer, and informal support groups. There is a memorial service twice a year for the staff and patients' families. Our five-year-old music therapy program visits patients at the hospital and at home.

 ### Education

Fellow and Resident Training

- *Fellowship in palliative medicine.*

This one-year clinical fellowship trains physicians in palliative medicine; board certification in another discipline is required (Le Grand et al., 2000). We may extend the fellowship to a second year if appropriate. Research is an essential part of the fellowship, which the Cleveland Clinic Foundation supports.

- *Fellowships.* All medical oncology and gynecological oncology fellows do a mandatory one-month rotation with the Palliative Medicine Program.
- *Internal medicine residents.* We are teaching the American Medical Association's Education of Physicians in End-of-Life-Care (EPEC) curriculum to the internal medicine residents. Internal medicine and family practice residents may elect rotations with the palliative medicine inpatient unit or the home hospice service.

Grand Rounds and Lectures

Palliative medicine participates in internal medicine training and internal medicine grand rounds, in addition to our own educational activities.

Roxane Scholars in Palliative Medicine

This program, funded by a pharmaceutical company (Roxane Laboratories, Columbus, Ohio), allows physicians, nurses, and

Table 2: Full Time Equivalents (FTEs) Supported by Clinical Revenue (1999–2000)

PALLIATIVE MEDICINE PROGRAM (1999–2000)	FTE	HOSPICE OF THE CLEVELAND CLINIC HOSPICE OFFICE	FTE
Attending physicians	4	Clinical chaplain	1
Clinical fellows	3	Administrative coordinator	1
Secretaries	3	Coordinator volunteers	1
Physician assistants	3	HIM coordinator	1
Medical social worker	1	Clinical manager	2
Nurse Clinician	2	Referral RN	1
Total	16	Pastoral care/bereavement coordinator	1
		Reimbursement specialist	1
		Hospice director	1
PALLIATIVE MEDICINE INPATIENT UNIT		Intake clerk	1
Registered nurses	18.2	Clerical	0.5
Unit secretary	2.5	Medical director	0.5
Assistant nurse manager	1	Total Office	12
Nurse manager	1	FIELD STAFF	
Licensed practical nurse	1.4	Registered nurse—full-time	8.5
Nursing unit assistants	8.4	Social worker—full-time	4
Total	32.50	Home health aides	9
		Other—part-time staff	5.5
		Total Field Staff	27.0
		Total Hospice	39.0
		TOTAL:	87.5

pharmacists to visit the Palliative Medicine Program for five days. The scholars see the program's day-to-day activities, make rounds with the inpatient and consultation teams, and sit in on all team meetings. In addition the scholars participate in educational activities.

Conferences

We incorporate educational conferences into the program's schedule. These include:

- *Grand rounds.* This weekly one-hour meeting reviews a syllabus for palliative medicine. A portion is also devoted to program development and monitoring program activities, for example, hospice staff meeting.
- *Research meeting.* At this weekly multidisciplinary meeting, we discuss new research ideas and projects and review the progress of current projects.
- *Morning report.* This is a daily update on clinical activities during the previous 24 hours. It summarizes the status of patients under the primary care of the program, gives information about new consults referred to the program, and coordinates hospital discharge planning. Interdisciplinary attendees represent hospice, home care, and case management.
- *Interdisciplinary team meeting.* This weekly one-hour meeting summarizes the clinical activities of the previous

week. It includes brief updates on community activity, research, and educational programs.

- *Hospice team meeting.* This weekly meeting, required by Medicare guidelines, is an interdisciplinary educational forum for clinical fellows and for residents in home and hospice care.
- *Weekly teaching.* This session with one of the attending physicians immediately follows morning report to ensure maximum attendance.
- *Problem case conference.* At this weekly meeting, a clinical case that poses particular difficulties for the hospital inpatient service is discussed in detail.
- *Journal report.* One of the clinical fellows presents a recent journal article at this weekly meeting, which the fellows direct.
- *Weekly case conference.* Fellows also direct meetings where they present interesting or controversial clinical, psychosocial, or ethical issues raised by a new patient referred to the program. Issues may concern management, symptom control, or medical complications.

Research

The need for research in palliative medicine is obvious. There are major deficiencies in our knowledge about the management of many common problems regarding symptoms, medical complications, and psychosocial issues. Kristine Nelson, M.D., research consultant to the program, has said: "Most of our research is patient-oriented and is easily and rapidly translated to clinical care. This immediate impact on patient care means that we are not only giving the care but also changing the care."

Under our research program we have a research attending physician. This is a full-time position dedicated to long-term strategy for research in palliative medicine, focusing primarily on symptom control. We also have two positions for research fellows to work with the research attending. The fellows train people interested in palliative medicine in clinical and research techniques. They develop a body of published work to further their careers. These activities complement research by the clinical fellows, who focus chiefly on patient care.

The main areas of research are: anorexia cachexia syndrome; common symptoms like pain and nausea; important drugs; nutritional assessment; management of common complications; psychosocial care; and quality of life.

In the future, we will seek long-term grants to aid our clinical research. We are also interested in the methodology of research, as there are significant practical, ethical, and humanitarian problems involved in conducting research into advanced disease. The traditional literature has not adequately addressed these problems, although they have inhibited progress in palliative care.

Lessons Learned

A number of lessons have emerged from program development since 1987.

Quality of Care
The first and most important lesson is that a relentless attention to the quality of patient care is the key to success. This focus must be reflected in every aspect of the program, from its broad-based clinical approach to research and education.

Academic Endeavor
The commitment to research and education is important not only for academic purposes but because it helps make excellence part of the program's culture.

Institutional Commitment
People who want to develop new Palliative Care programs frequently emphasize that they will save money. This is a zero sum option: in reviewing proposals for new programs, the simplest administrative response is to say no and thereby avoid risk.

This is particularly true of any financial commitment to a program of uncertain future and debatable benefit to an organization. It is also difficult to prove that a palliative medicine program will actually save money, given the vagaries of health care financing and accounting practices. Furthermore the fiscal argument can doom the new program to eternal downsizing, just to survive. This is incompatible with program growth. Growth requires investment of resources, long-term development of personnel, and a serious commitment by the parent organization to initiating and maintaining a vibrant new clinical program.

Businesslike Approach

Focus on the value added to the organization through better clinical care, earlier discharge from the hospital, positive community image, and increased philanthropic donations for humanitarian clinical activities.

Personnel

In health care program development, adequate resources are not allocated unless it is clear that the program's personnel and resources are overcommitted. This is particularly hazardous to a new program. Capable individuals may burn out from the relentless overload needed in order to expand the program. The inevitable stress will cause staff attrition in the process of achieving the otherwise laudable goals of program development.

Marketing

Never promote a service or program unless you are committed to, and confident of, successful delivery.

Postacute Care Services: The Future of Palliative Medicine?

Any health system should be responsible for effective and timely discharge planning. This is central to the financial well-being of every hospital in the United States. The issues of case management, discharge planning, and continuity of high-quality medical care in the hospital, the outpatient clinic, the rehabilitation unit, the subacute unit, the nursing home, and the various home care services is an important part of this process. As the population ages rapidly over the next two decades, postacute care will become even more important. Providing this care as patients flow from postacute care to acute care and back again, will be a significant part of the health care business, clinically and financially.

Palliative medicine at the Cleveland Clinic Foundation is deeply involved in both acute and postacute care, which makes it an unusual medical discipline. The important

role that palliative medicine plays in
continuity of care as patients with life-limiting
illness cycle between the hospital and the
community qualifies it to monitor other
clinical services with similar design and intent.
Health systems may want to keep the money
from postacute services within their own
province. That is the major clinical incentive
for a seamless, multidisciplinary continuum of
services. Palliative medicine is uniquely suited
to participate in the design, management, and
medical leadership of that continuum.

Patient Population (1998)

On any given day, the program follows about 240 patients, about half of whom are on the home hospice service. The median age of our patients is 65. The predominant diagnosis is cancer, distributed almost exactly like the major causes of cancer mortality nationwide. A significant number of patients are immigrants from eastern Europe.

CONSULTS

Total:		834
Inpatient	505	
Outpatient	329	
(Hematology/Oncology	*294)*	
Weekly Average		16
Inpatient	10	
Outpatient	6	

ACTIVE CENSUS

Weekly Average		200
Palliative Medicine	115	
Hospice	85	

INPATIENT ADMISSIONS

Total:		633
Weekly Average:	12	
PCS Primary	2	
Hospice	3	
New to PCS	3	

INPATIENT CENSUS

Daily Average:		17
Primary	13	
Hospice	2	

SCHEDULED OUTPATIENT VISITS

Total:		1,374
Weekly Average:		26

DEATHS

Total:		541
Palliative Medicine	157	
Hospice	186	
Horvitz Center	140	
Palliative Home Care	58	
Weekly Average:		11
Palliative Medicine	3	
Hospice	4	
Horvitz Center	3	
Palliative Home Care	1	

Hospice of the Cleveland Clinic, January 1–December 31, 1998

TOTAL REFERRALS:	833			**VISITS:**		
				Nursing:	8,628	35%
TOTAL STARTS OF CARE:	550			Social work:	2,327	9%
Referral Source				Home health aide:	11,643	47%
CCF:	502	91%		Pastoral care:	1,711	7%
Metro:	12	2%		LPN:	470	1%
Ventures:	36	6%		Physical therapy:	82	<1%
				Physical therapy assistant:	21	<1%
AVERAGE DAILY CENSUS:	87			Occupational therapy:	11	<1%
				Speech therapy:	4	<1%
SEX:				Medical director:	30	<1%
Male:	269	49%		Total:	24,927	
Female:	281	51%				

ETHNICITY:

White:	391	71%	**ROUTINE HOME CARE DAYS**	
Black:	109	20%	**"PER DIEM":**	33,533
Unknown:	40	7%	Payers (per diem days):	
Hispanic:	3	1%	Medicare:	19,558
Asian:	4	1%	Blue Cross:	3,741
American Indian:	3	1%	Medicaid:	951
			Aetna:	2,552
DIAGNOSES (TOP 5)			Emerald:	1,107
Lung Cancer:	147		Self-Pay:	3,454
Colon Cancer:	47		Other Insurance:	2,170
Breast Cancer:	32			
Pancreatic Cancer:	31		**AVERAGE LENGTH OF STAY:**	55
Brain Cancer:	25		(Total per diem days/total per diem patients)	

TOTAL DEATHS: 505

Home:	298	59%	**TOTAL NUMBER OF GENERAL**
Hospital:	32	6%	**INPATIENT DAYS:** 452
Other Nursing Home:	28	5%	(Hospice-related)
Inpatient Hospice Facility:	147	29%	

**INPATIENT DAYS IN RELATION TO TOTAL
OF PER DIEM ROUTINE HOME CARE DAYS
(RELATED ADMISSIONS):** 1%

The Harry R. Horvitz Center for Palliative
Medicine, The Cleveland Clinic Foundation
Funding Sources, January 1 — December 31, 1998*

Medicare	58%	■
Other Insurance	30%	■
Personal Pay	9%	■
Medicaid	3%	■

*Percentages have been rounded off.

REFERENCES

Ahmedzai, S., and D. Walsh. 2000 Palliative Medicine and Modern Cancer Care. *Seminars in Oncology*, 27(1):1–6.

Goldstein, P., D. Walsh, and L. Horvitz. 1996. The Cleveland Clinic Foundation Harry R. Horvitz Palliative Care Center. *Supportive Care in Cancer*, 4:329–33.

LeGrand, S.B., D. Walsh, K.N. Nelson, and D.S. Zhukovsky. 2000. Development of a Clinical Fellowship Program in Palliative Medicine. *Journal of Pain and Symptom Management*, in press.

Miller, R.D., R. Krech, and T.D. Walsh. 1991. The Role of a Palliative Care Service Family Conference in the Management of the Patient with Advanced Cancer. *Palliative Medicine*, 5:34–9.

Miller, R., and T.D. Walsh. 1991. Psychosocial Aspects of Palliative Care in Advanced Cancer. *Journal of Pain and Symptom Management*, 6(1):24–9.

Nelson, K., D. Walsh, O. Abdullah, et al. 2000a. Common Complications of Advanced Cancer. *Seminars in Oncology*, 27(1):34–44.

Nelson, K., D. Walsh, C. Behrens, D. Zhukovsky, V. Lipnickey, and D. Brady. 2000b. The Dying Cancer Patient. *Seminars in Oncology*, 27(1):84–9.

Stagno, S., D. Zhukovsky, and D. Walsh. 2000. Bioethics: Communication and Decision Making in Advanced Disease. *Seminars in Oncology*, 27(1)94–100.

Tropiano, P., D. Zajac, and D. Walsh. 2000. Organization of Services and Nursing Care: Hospice and Palliative Medicine. *Seminars in Oncology*, 27(1):7–13.

Walsh, D. 1990. Continuing Care in a Medical Center: The Cleveland Clinic Foundation Palliative Care Service. *Journal of Pain and Symptom Management*, 5(5): 273–8.

Walsh, D. 1994a. Palliative Care: Management of the Patient with Advanced Cancer. *Seminars in Oncology*, 21(4): 100–6.

Walsh, D., W. Gombeski, P. Goldstein, D. Hayes, and M. Armour. 1994b. Managing a Palliative Oncology Program: The Role of a Business Plan. *Journal of Pain and Symptom Management,* 9(2):109–18.

Walsh, D. 1997. Symptom Control in Advanced Cancer. Proceedings of the 33rd Annual Meeting of the American Society of Clinical Oncology; Denver, Colo. 295–302.

Walsh, D. 1998. The Medicare Hospice Benefit: A Critique from Palliative Medicine. *Journal of Palliative Medicine,* 1(2):147–9.

Walsh, D., M. Doona, M. Molnar, and V. Lipnickey. 2000. Symptom Control in Advanced Cancer: Important Drugs and Routes of Administration. *Seminars in Oncology,* 27(1):69–83.

Massachusetts General Hospital Palliative Care Service

J. Andrew Billings

Inspiration and Motivation

I became interested in palliative care after stumbling into home care in 1975. That year, I finished my house staff training at the University of California, San Francisco, and took a job as a physician at the Massachusetts General Hospital–Chelsea Memorial Health Center, a neighborhood health center in a poor, multi-ethnic community a few miles—and seemingly a whole world—away from MGH. My predecessor at the health center, a British general practitioner working in the United States for a year, had followed a few elderly patients at home. On my first day, she suggested that I visit two patients who were being cared for at home by devoted relatives. I had never made a house call, but I immediately enjoyed the adventure and began to visit patients' houses regularly. Members of a multidisciplinary team at MGH supported my work with homebound patients; this team was composed of doctors, nurses, a social worker, a geriatric outreach worker, a nutritionist, and a medical librarian, who met to talk about complicated geriatric cases, usually focusing on the home care cases. While my medical colleagues may have thought I was a bit odd at times, they also saw the value of house calls, and many of them related warm stories of their own experiences with home care.

Many families in Chelsea and nearby communities had cared for a sick relative at home, and many patients expected to be cared for at home until the end of their lives. Indeed, my first two patients were elderly and demented. One was cared for by a spouse, the other by a son, and both of them died at home. I learned from my patients, their families, and some of my colleagues—particularly nurses and social workers—about caring for sick people, especially the terminally ill, at home. One of my physician-mentors gave a talk on caring for dying people at home, alerting me to some of the intellectual challenges of this work and suggesting ways for me to train others about key tasks.

Around 1978, an acquaintance who knew of my interest in home care asked me to join a planning group, inspired by the work of Cicely Saunders, founder of St. Christopher's Hospice in London, that eventually led to the first hospice program in Massachusetts. I was its medical director and, later, president of the organization. I began studying more about terminal care, visited St. Christopher's, and attended conferences given by the Hospice of New Haven, the National Hospice Organization, and Balfour Mount, founder of the Palliative Care Service at Montreal's Royal Victoria Hospital. I began practicing and teaching about end-of-life care, particularly about pain and symptom management and about helping families care for the dying at home, and I wrote a book on the subject, *Outpatient Management of Advanced Cancer: Symptom Control, Support and Hospice-in-the-Home*. At about that time, I developed a proposal to create a palliative care service at Massachusetts General Hospital and shared it with a few colleagues, but I never pursued the matter.

After a merger and collapse of our volunteer hospice program in the early 1980s, I spent a few years concentrating on medical education and teaching clinical interviewing as part of the New Pathway project at Harvard Medical School. I completed a book on clinical interviewing. I developed a number of teaching modules on end-of-life issues, and acquired new notions about pedagogy, the hospital culture, and the need for institutional change.

Around 1987, I got re-involved with hospice when Jo Magno invited me to speak at an early meeting of the International Hospice Institute. I participated in the founding of the Academy of Hospice Physicians (now the American Academy of Hospice and Palliative Medicine) and served as a board member and president. I was pleased to have the opportunity to meet and work with Balfour Mount, Eduardo Bruera, and Neil MacDonald from Edmonton, and a host of United States clinicians interested in palliative care. I helped develop this group's

teaching programs and newsletter. In Boston, I was invited to participate in the development of Trinity Hospice, an inner-city hospice program with ties to local academic hospitals, and I became its medical director. Part of this hospice's mission was to bring the hospice philosophy to training institutions. I also became the national medical director for a large home care company, and had the opportunity to start a number of hospices and to train their medical directors.

Up to this point, practically all my work as a palliative care physician and educator was conducted outside of a hospital or medical school. As medical director for Trinity Hospice, however, I developed relationships with many oncologists at Massachusetts General Hospital. I also became more interested in creating programs that would let house officers and fellows learn about good end-of-life care and that would extend the hospice approach to academic centers. When I later learned about the Faculty Scholars Program of the Project on Death in America (PDIA), I decided to prepare a proposal for a program in palliative care at MGH. The grant from PDIA gave me the courage to give up some of my regular clinical work and to focus on developing a Palliative Care Service. Declan Walsh of the Cleveland Clinic and Balfour Mount were particularly helpful at this stage in planning the Service.

Peddling my dream program, I found many supporters in all parts of the hospital. When I had first become involved in hospice, nobody knew what the word meant. By the late 1980s, however, the medical community had become more knowledgeable about hospice and generally thought of it as a good thing. Disenchantment with current end-of-life care was widespread. In this environment, the idea of a hospice-like service was quickly grasped and favorably regarded by many administrators and clinicians at MGH.

By January 1997, when we opened the MGH Palliative Care Service, hardly anyone knew what "palliative care" meant. I did a lot of explaining. But today the new house staff that arrives each year sees the Service as an established part of MGH. The Service quickly became known and accepted, at least within the medical service and in oncology, where we focused our initial efforts.

I continue to find my encounters with patients and families tremendously exciting and rewarding. I am repeatedly struck by the intensity of their needs, the frequency of untended problems, my ability to help them quickly, their gratitude and lessened anxiety, and my effectiveness in making personal contact and providing comfort. I love the opportunity to learn about their lives, and I continue to appreciate the authenticity and intimacy that can characterize the doctor-patient relationship. Palliative care allows me to use my clinical skills best, to be effective in helping patients and families, to educate other clinicians, and to be the kind of physician and person I strive to be. I believe that every case is a "good case." As difficult patient and family situations are presented to me, I keep finding myself saying, "Isn't that interesting?" or "We're going to learn something different here." We always seem to make a substantial contribution to the care of the patient and family.

Unfortunately, much of my current work is administrative, and it is much less gratifying than direct patient care. I must now welcome my role in helping others learn about and give good end-of-life care. I have developed a number of programs that allow me to teach about this subject, and I relish this teaching. I hope that my students will go on to give good care and share my pleasure in this field.

I also greatly enjoy the multidisciplinary team we have assembled. We had chosen a multidisciplinary team from the beginning and were able to add staff, including an additional half-time physician, as the service became more established. I am grateful for my colleagues' fine work and for their stimulating and supportive companionship. While I have always savored medicine and found the daily clinical encounters with patients and families stimulating and gratifying, I do not believe I have ever delighted in my work, including my professional relationships, as much as I do now.

If I could have done one thing differently, I would have started the program with another physician or team of physicians or would have set some limits on my availability. In the beginning, I was the only physician on our team, and I was on call all the time. As a matter of principle, and to maintain the Service's public image within the hospital, I felt that our service had to be available at all times and that we needed to make rounds on our patients daily, including weekends. While having full personal responsibility for the program certainly has some advantages, I would have preferred not to have been on call every weekend. Night calls were rare, but the burden of working every weekend was great. I would have benefited from a colleague who could cross-cover. In retrospect, I might have closed the Service on weekends.

 Program Development

. . . .

The goal of the Palliative Care Service is to provide comprehensive, continuing, coordinated, interdisciplinary services to terminally ill patients and their families and to be a center of academic excellence and training in care at the end of life. While our work is based on the hospice model and is devoted to dying people and their families, we believe that palliative care is essential to

good care at all phases of life. We do not subscribe to the artificial separation of hospice methods from other aspects of care.

The original plan for the Service was to establish an inpatient consultation service, an outpatient program integrated with a home hospice program, and an inpatient palliative care unit, and eventually to develop alternative institutional sites of care. We anticipated that the outpatient practice would be much larger than the inpatient one.

When the Service was proposed, the hospital was gearing up for managed care and consolidation of medical services in the region. A key administrator with considerable expertise in hospice inpatient units expected to close many beds and was unsympathetic to the notion of a dedicated inpatient palliative care unit, which seemed to glamorize hospital-based services instead of fostering outpatient care. Consequently, we had to put our plan for the inpatient palliative care unit on hold, though it was not abandoned. I had designed an integrated combination of inpatient and home-hospice care in collaboration with a hospice, but that hospice collapsed, quashing my formal alliance with a hospice. (This sort of collaboration with hospice has been proposed repeatedly over the past few years, but has only recently begun to look like a real possibility.) Regardless of these setbacks, the hospital's focus on fiscal performance produced great enthusiasm for a program that promised to reduce ancillaries on a very expensive group of inpatients, promote early discharge, and help patients stay at home, while teaching house staff habits of restraint in the use of expensive technology at the end of life. We also suggested that we might draw new patients into our network.

Key Steps in the Development of the Program

This is one recipe for developing a palliative care service.

- Be a solid citizen. I was recognized by at least some of the MGH leadership and staff as a dedicated and skilled clinician and teacher.

- Have a great product. Palliative care is the right idea at about the right time.

- Write a strong prospectus that is brief but engaging, and present it with enthusiasm and skill. I talked about the program wherever someone would listen to me. I got on the agenda of any committee that might be interested in this program, then presented it with care, enthusiasm, and respect for the committee's questions and concerns.

- Comb the hospital for potential supporters, particularly among the leadership, and promote the program to them in various ways. This step was relatively easy, since everyone seemed to

like the program, though many people had reservations about its cost. I talked to every hospital leader who might be vital to the administrative acceptance of the program. Surprisingly, some of its most important supporters, who were preoccupied with the disagreeable task of closing beds and cutting costs, were pleased to be working for a program that was a "good thing to do." Fortunately, I obtained early support from a key administrator who designated an excellent assistant to serve as my administrator, directed me to important decision makers, helped us strategize, and eventually pushed the program through various administrative potholes.

- Have chutzpah. I felt the project was important enough to deserve the attention of everyone in the hospital, and I made sure that it got the attention it deserved.

- Get funding. My PDIA fellowship made the project financially possible.

- Prepare a detailed fiscal analysis of the impact of the program, and then help the fiscal department to understand it and translate it into a format with which the department is familiar.

Barriers to Program Development

Aside from fiscal matters, I think I was much more aware of the potential problems with developing the Service than any of the hospital leaders were. They seemed to accept that the Service was desirable as long as it did not cost much, and my job was to talk to them about the necessity for the program and to assure them that it was financially sound. Other forms of resistance that I anticipated seemed to become important only after we opened the program and looked for referrals.

These issues arose after the program had been in operation for a couple of months. Now they seem to be part of our daily work:

- Services protect their turf. Sometimes Oncology or the Pain Service feels it should do the work.

- A new service may affect education or patterns of clinical practice. That is, palliative care may draw dying patients into non-teaching programs or move them out of the regular wards into an isolated spot. Clinicians may have abandoned dying patients or may become less skilled in terminal care because they refer dying patients to the Palliative Care Service.

- Some may view palliative care as physician-assisted suicide. Muddled ideas about the "double effect" of painkillers or the ethical implications of withholding or withdrawing care must be combated.

- When clinicians hear that end-of-life care is inadequate, they interpret it as criticism. Primary care physicians with whom I had worked for years felt that they could do just as good a job as I.

The Service quickly took off as an inpatient consultation team, leaving me little time to make house calls or see nursing home patients. Moreover, unlike my work in the community-based practice or the inner-city hospice services, the work here included many patients who lived great distances from the hospital. We were involved with discharge planning and supervised some care in the home, but we usually relied on the visiting nurses or hospice team to make house calls and had to become familiar with the availability and quality of services throughout the greater Boston area. We even played a significant role in the management of patients in Venezuela and Mexico.

Our ability to provide hospice-like care to non-hospice patients was very attractive to many physicians, especially oncologists, who had had bad experiences with one or more hospices that had refused to admit patients who needed expensive palliative treatments (e.g., radiation or parenteral nutrition). At times, our unfamiliar name was advantageous; people with negative views on hospice had not had time to form negative opinions of palliative care!

Most of the physicians who referred hospital patients to us, and who wanted our help with discharge planning and outpatient management, preferred to continue being responsible for these patients when they returned to the hospital. Very few of the patients we discharged or saw in the community ever returned to the hospital. Therefore, we have primary responsibility for few inpatients, and we function largely as consultants on the inpatient wards.

Changes in the hospice community, including frequent turnover of leadership and the resulting administrative instability, made it difficult to establish good working relationships with hospices. Consequently, the Service now consists mainly of inpatient consultation at the MGH and the Spaulding Rehabilitation Hospital nearby, and a little outpatient visiting, home care, and nursing-home care.

In obtaining initial approval and support from the hospital, I was fortunate to identify many allies. A few administrators and department heads who appreciated both the benefits of hospice and my work helped me through the process. I also garnered support from a great number of leaders from all parts of MGH. This process, however, was very time consuming. The money from PDIA helped, by giving me the time I needed and by signaling hospital personnel that the project had been endorsed.

But when the Service actually opened, the support from hospital leaders was less helpful than I expected. Some of the social workers and discharge planners I had worked with, who had always clearly supported palliative care, seemed unenthused about making referrals to the Service and hung on to many patients the Service would have liked to see. Nurses generally responded very positively to the Service but played a lesser role in generating referrals. Physicians generally seemed to appreciate our work but referred patients to the Service only when a strong need emerged, typically in unusually difficult cases. Oncologists quickly became familiar with our service, and we rely heavily on these "satisfied customers" for our referrals.

Another surprise is that patients are rarely referred for pain and symptom problems, though many of our patients have these problems and we regularly work on symptom management. The hospital has had a Pain Service for many years, and that service, rather than ours, is usually called when a pain problem arises, even if the patient is terminally ill. The Pain Service initially was worried that our interest in pain would lead to their losing patients. I have partially countered this fear by befriending the leaders of the Pain Service and striving vigorously to cooperate with them, finding opportunities for joint training of house staff and fellows, having our staff attend their cancer pain rounds, and developing a joint project with them to teach pain assessment and management throughout the hospital.

Our most effective marketing strategy—call it serendipity—was doing a research program on three wards of the Medical Service. Once the medical house staff got to know us, they began using us almost routinely. I look for opportunities to make the Palliative Care Service visible in the daily life of the hospital's professional staff. We continue to look for opportunities to familiarize the hospital staff with our work by orienting staff, conducting grand rounds, getting publicity in the hospital newsletter, and the like.

My major worry right now is that the Service does not readily pay for itself from clinical revenues. We justified our Service partly on the basis of cost offsets, which are hard to prove. We have had significant difficulties with billing. We have arranged for many of our expenses to be covered by the hospital, rather than by the physicians' organization that receives our clinical billing. We have done this for two reasons: (1) because the kind of care we provide is very time consuming, reimbursement is very poor relative to the time involved, and (2) much of the care we provide, including the services of the nurse, social worker, and chaplain, is not reimbursable at all.

I have also offset much of my own salary and some staff salary by obtaining grants. We are looking for other grants and donations that might help assure our survival. For now, I think that our expenses are small enough so that the good will and endorsement from hospital leaders and our continuing favorable publicity will keep us going.

I think the Service could function fairly well without me, since I have a very competent associate physician and interdisciplinary team. I think our reputation would sustain us and allow us to grow, and I think the staff would carry out our mission appropriately. However, leadership remains important, particularly for interacting with the hospital administration and heads of other services, developing new initiatives, and maintaining a balance between programmatic and fiscal goals. Because the main barrier to our long-term success appears to be fiscal, I have been very active in seeking help from the MGH Development Office and in finding grants to support our activities.

We have not been aggressive marketers. For most of the Service's history, we have been struggling to keep up with our caseload. Our emphasis has been on providing good care and helping our colleagues in their work, not on getting more referrals. We have also emphasized teaching others to do the work rather than abrogating care to our team, though I presume that any effort to promote higher standards of practice in end-of-life care will not only help many patients we never see but will also lead to referrals of more difficult cases. For example, during our first two years, a few members of our team attended weekly multidisciplinary rounds on the inpatient oncology floor and played a significant role in reviewing difficult cases with its nurses and social workers. This led to good working relationships, more awareness on the floor of the value of chaplaincy, more appreciation of the role of staff support, and some referrals.

One exception to our low-key approach is a highly visible pain relief initiative, which is administered jointly with the pain service and nursing. Here we have sought a lot of publicity but have not focused on our Service. We have also been active in many formal and informal efforts to improve end-of-life care by consulting with or joining various committees and community groups and by conducting teaching sessions. For instance, both Service physicians and our fellow are on the hospital ethics committee, which concentrates almost exclusively on end-of-life care, and my associate physician led efforts to write a new set of hospital-wide guidelines about ethics in terminal illness. Our nurse practitioner has played a role in community efforts to promote good end-of-life care and to form a coalition of

organizations in Massachusetts that might attract funding. I worked briefly with the state medical association and with the legislature on related issues.

Institutional Culture

Hindrances

Institutional culture can impede palliative care.

- The house staff and some physicians tend to focus on making a precise diagnosis and offering aggressive treatment in situations in which, I believe, more appropriate care might involve tolerating diagnostic uncertainty. Our Service is less preoccupied with getting all the data and pinning down a diagnosis, especially when we feel a precise diagnosis would not affect the patient's treatment, or when the morbidity of a procedure does not seem appropriate or worthwhile.

- Physicians and other staff may overlook the informed wishes of patients and families.

- Staff may ask the patient and family to choose treatment options, including use of cardiopulmonary resuscitation, without appropriate guidance.

- Comprehensive, interdisciplinary services, including psychosocial and spiritual care, may be lacking in some settings or be lost as patients transfer from one institution to another or to home.

- The staff may be unfamiliar with the potential for providing excellent care at home, may overvalue the hospital, and may underestimate how conventional inpatient care contributes to suffering.
- The hospital tends to change very slowly.
- Fiscal crises caused all hospital programs to be carefully scrutinized for their cost. No program can be a financial drain on the hospital. Hiring was occasionally frozen, and new programs were the first to be cut. By being aware of this focus on finances and providing detailed fiscal analyses, I was able to surmount this barrier and even turn it to our advantage at times.

Program Support

The personal support of the senior administrator on the Medical Service was invaluable to the Palliative Care Service's ability to get and keep institutional support. Given the go-ahead by the chief of the Medical Service, she appointed an excellent, hard-driving associate to get the project going. She worked with a number of leaders in the Medical Service and hospital administration, who coached our team repeatedly. When the project proposal got lost in the Fiscal Department or languished on someone's desk, the top administrator repeatedly helped move it along. More recently, in expanding parts of the program

and improving the appearance of our balance sheets by shifting costs to the hospital, a trustee and fund-raiser has been essential in encouraging the president of MGH to support the Service. Also vital to the program's success was support from, among others, the chief of General Internal Medicine, administrators in the Department of Medicine, and a senior administrator in the Cancer Center.

The fact that our program has a group of talented, engaging, hard-working clinicians who are committed to the goals of the Palliative Care Service has also been critical to its success.

I. Institutional Information

    A.   Name of program: Massachusetts General Hospital Palliative Care Service

    B.   Program director: J. Andrew Billings, MD

    C.   Program start date: January 1997

    D.   Institutional setting: Urban

    E.   Type of institution: Academic hospital with affiliated network, medical school, and residency training

    F.   Number of beds: about 750

    G.   Health care system

        1. Hospital affiliates: one major affiliate nearby and about 7 more distant affiliates

        2. Long-term care affiliates: at least 2

II. Program Characteristics

    A.   Direct Service Staff

        1.   Physicians: 2 half-time generalists, one with a PhD in philosophy and advanced training in general internal medicine and ethics

        2.   Nurses: 1 full-time nurse practitioner with specialized training in cancer and extensive experience with hospice

        3.   Social worker: 1 full-time social worker with background in hospice, pediatric oncology, and adult care

        4.   Other providers: full-time chaplain/bereavement coordinator

    B.   Research Staff

        1.   Dedicated staff: only on grants

        2.   One nurse–project director full-time for pain initiative; 2.5 FTE (full-time equivalents) to be hired soon on a palliative care education grant. Also, a full-time physician-researcher on one earlier project, a half-time research assistant on a recently completed study, and a full-time researcher on a new project

    C.   Administrative Staff

        Full-time administrative assistant for our Service and a part-time administrator from the Medical Service, plus lots of occasional helpers from various parts of the hospital, including the development office

    D.   Clinical Characteristics

        1.   Part of the General Internal Medicine Unit of the Medical Services

2. Primarily an inpatient consultation service with some primary care services and limited outpatient/home care/hospice service

3. No dedicated inpatient unit

4. No formally affiliated, dedicated inpatient hospice unit

5. Formally affiliated home hospice program is about to be created

6. Formally affiliated home-care program is about to be created

E. Patient Population

    1. No inpatient unit

    2. Monthly inpatient consultations: 36 (mean 6.54 days to discharge or death; median 4.6)

    3. Monthly patients receiving home care: 112, including hospice (mean 25.4 days to death; median 30.2 days)

    4. Monthly patients receiving hospice care: 60

F. Demographics (see box)

G. Funding

    1. Foundation grants: 0.55 FTE MD and 0.7 FTE fellow

    2. Federal grants 0.28 FTE MD

    3. Endowments

    4. Charity

    5. Hospital support: nurse, social worker, chaplain/bereavement coordinator, rent and utilities, and 0.5 FTE physician

    6. Medical school support: none

    7. Clinical income: 0.4 FTE physician and 0.3 FTE fellow

H. Educational Component and Outside Funding (no funding unless noted)

    1. Fellows from pain, anesthesia, medicine, oncology, etc. rotate on Service electively

    2. Residents rotate on Service electively

    3. Medical students

        a. one-term elective course (2 hours of class time per week) supported by NCI grant

        b. elective rotations

        c. summer and year-long research assistants with various outside funding

    4. Faculty/Colleagues

        a. Fellowship in palliative care, one year

Demographics of Palliative Care Service Patient Population

			3.	DISPOSITION

1. **DIAGNOSES (1998)**

Cancer	86%
Congestive heart failure	6%
Neurologic	5%
Other	3%

2. **AGE (1998)**

0-24	1%
25-44	9%
45-64	32%
65+	58%

3. **DISPOSITION**
- Discharged to home: 57%
- Died in hospital: 43%
- Died in chronic care or nursing home: 20%
- Referred to hospice or home care: about 15-20 per month
- Referred to hospice: 63% of those dying at home
- Referred to conventional home care: 37% of those dying at home

In the first 7 months of FY1999, 1,047 charges were submitted for a total of $89,960, which would project to charges of about $154,000 per year.

ACCOUNTS RECEIVABLE, 1999

Blue Shield	11%
HMOs	18%
Commercial	5%
Medicare	55%
Medicaid	10%
Self-Pay	2%

AVERAGE MONTHLY REFERRALS

	1997	1998	1999
Inpatient	16	18	28
Specialty Rehabilitation	2	3	4
Outpatient	2	2	3

AVERAGE MONTHLY HOME CARE POPULATION

1997	55
1998	85
1999	102

SITE OF DEATH

	NUMBER	PERCENT
MGH	98	43%
Chronic care/Nursing home	45	20%
Palliative care unit	18	8%
Home*	65	29%
TOTAL	**226**	**100%**

* 63% deaths in home-hospice care, 37% in conventional home care.

1999 AVERAGE MONTHLY FIGURES

	INPATIENT*	HOME CARE#
Total days/mos	244	2715
Mean length of stay/mos	6.54	25.41
Median length of stay/mos	4.6	30.2

* Inpatient figures are for time until death or discharge.

Home care figures are for time until death or admission to an institution.

b. Palliative care grand rounds weekly and multiple presentations at teaching conferences

c. Visiting programs, usually 1–2 days

d. Palliative Care Role Model Program for 16 faculty each year, supported by NCI grant

e. Palliative Care Education Program for nurses and physicians entails 14 days a year on site, supported by the Robert Wood Johnson Foundation

5. Nurses supervised in nurse-practitioner training

6. Social workers supervised in training placements

7. Occasional public presentations

III. Research Component: Funding Sources

A. Percent federal grants: 40%

B. Percent foundation grants: 60%

C. Percent industry: 0

D. Percent intramural: 0

E. Current research projects (see list of active projects under "Grants," below)

MGH Palliative Care Service Revenue Sources, 1999*

Medicare	54%	■
HMOs	18%	▨
Blue Shield	11%	▨
Medicaid	10%	■
Commercial	5%	▨
Self-Pay	2%	■

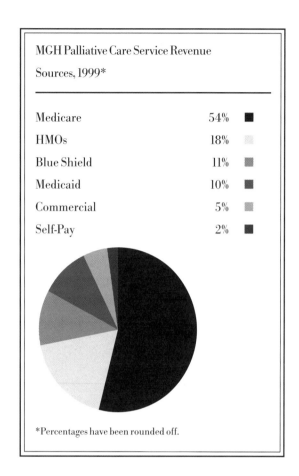

*Percentages have been rounded off.

PAST

(Block)   9/30/94–9/29/97

National Cancer Institute $161,477

Hospice in General Medical Education and Primary Care

Establishment of a new course at Harvard Medical School, "Living with Life Threatening Illness."

(Billings)   7/1/95–6/30/98

Project on Death in America $229,500

Faculty Scholar

This project is meant to develop a Palliative Care Service at the Massachusetts General Hospital,
including opportunities for clinical palliative care education for health profession students
and practitioners.

(Billings)   10/1/96–9/31/97

Milton Fund (Harvard University) $12,000

Care of the Dying in an Academic Medical Center

A randomized, controlled evaluation of a new palliative care service.

(Block)   1996–1997

Open Society Institute Project on Death in America $93,000

and The Robert Wood Johnson Foundation (#029360)

National Consensus Conference for Care Near the End of Life

A 2-day conference with workshops, involving a broad range of leaders in medical education,
leading to the development of a series of published consensus papers.

(Solomon)   6/1/96–5/31/2000

#R01 HS0869-01 $1,886,117

Agency for Health Care Policy and Research

Adoption of Cancer Pain Guidelines in Managed Care

This project aims to determine the two-tiered (organizational and individual) dissemination strategy on health care providers' adoption in a managed care setting of the AHCPR's cancer pain guidelines.

(McPeek)   9/1/96–5/31/99

ROI HS08691-03 $26,827 (sub only)

Agency for Health Care Policy and Research

Cancer Pain Relief in a Managed Care Setting

This project aims to determine the two-tiered (organizational and individual) dissemination strategy on health care providers' adoption in a managed care setting of the AHCPR's cancer pain guidelines.

(Block)   12/1/97–11/30/02

#R25 CA 66818 – 04 $423,349

National Cancer Institute Cancer Education

Palliative Care Role Model Program

This grant supports a faculty development program to train clinical leaders at three academic centers to be palliative care role models, clinicians, and educators.

(Billings)   7/1/98–9/31/00

Mayday Fund $257,000

"MGH Cares about Pain"

This grant supports a 27-month hospital-wide initiative to improve assessment and management of pain by clinical staff.

(Billings)   3/1/99–2/28/02

Robert Wood Johnson Foundation $997,874

Harvard Medical Center for Palliative Care Faculty Development Program

This grant supports a 3-year national center for training medical and nursing faculty about

palliative care clinical practice and educational methods.

(Tennstedt)   9/30/99–6/30/2000

R01 NR05154 $116,951 (subcontract)

National Institute of Nursing Research

Advanced Stage Chronic Disease: Symptoms, Distress, Care

A study of the end-of-life distress of patients with chronic lung and heart disease.

(Billings)

Ortho-Biotech   7/1/99–6/31/00

Palliative Care Fellowship $65,000

One-year funding for a fellow.

(Billings)

National Cancer Institute   7/1/01–6/30/05

Palliative Care Fellowship $869,356

Funding to establish a fellowship at the Massachusetts General Hospital that provides a broad

background in palliative care clinical practice as well as expertise in educating others about this

field. The fellowship will evolve into a 2-year program with research training.

Palliative Care Program
Medical College of Virginia Campus of
Virginia Commonwealth University

Laurel J. Lyckholm, Patrick J. Coyne, and Thomas J. Smith

Overview

The MCV-VCU Palliative Care Program has been in development since 1994. It formally began with the opening of the Thomas Hospice Palliative Care Unit in May 2000. The goal of this program is to bring compassionate care to those who are dying throughout central Virginia and to improve access for medically underserved people.

In 1994, Patrick Coyne and Thomas J. Smith identified palliative care as a major deficiency of our academic health center. As we expanded our care of cancer and AIDS patients, we simply got tired of their having nowhere to go to die. We decided to fix the problem. The hospital and cancer center agreed that the fourth-largest academic health care center in the United States should have comprehensive services, from diagnosis to cure or death. To demonstrate the need for a palliative care unit, we began to monitor the number of patients who needed such care by taking a weekly census of the dying patients who were hospitalized at MCV-VCU Hospitals. We found a daily census of more than 25 people, six on oncology alone. In 1995, we performed a brief audit of 20 patients who had died in the hospital. The audit documented wide variations in the quality of care and the resources used. We found expensive, high-technology, unreimbursed care when low-tech caring was needed.

In 1996, we began negotiating with the hospital for space for a palliative care inpatient unit. We sought start-up funds from the Jessie Ball DuPont Fund, a charitable organization that supports community-based projects, which had been instrumental in helping us develop the Rural Cancer Outreach Program. We applied for and obtained a grant for almost $300,000 in 1997 (which was still sitting in the bank as of February 2000!). The outreach program had shown that we had the skills and entrepreneurial spirit to develop novel, highly visible programs that created good will and to use them to teach, improve care, and lower the total cost of care. More important, we could improve the bottom line of the academic hospital (Desch et al., 1992; Smith et al., 1991; Smith et al., 1996; Desch et al., 1999).

In 1997, the Thomas Hospice, a not-for-profit group based in Richmond, joined our program. It had begun Richmond's first hospice in 1971 at Retreat Hospital, a small urban hospital that was clinically successful and financially stable until Retreat was acquired by Columbia/HCA. Columbia/HCA closed the hospice, which did not meet the company's financial goals, leaving this community group with no physical home. The group tried to partner with the Bon Secours health system, a Catholic charitable organization that provides acute and chronic inpatient care throughout the mid-Atlantic region, but could not establish common goals and structure. The Thomas Hospice has provided us with administrative support, a community base, and education and training programs for hospice volunteers. In addition, Thomas provides substantial financial backing for the future. To start, Thomas put $100,000 on the table for renovations.

The period from 1997 to 1999 saw substantial delays in our program due to lack of appropriate inpatient space. It has taken more than two and a half years to relocate the occupants of the space, including psychiatry day programs, electroconvulsive therapy, and house staff offices, to different areas of the hospital or to space off campus.

The Thomas Hospice Palliative Care Unit opened in May 2000. It is an 11-bed inpatient unit with one "swing" bed used for procedures. It will be fully staffed for outpatient infusions and procedures as well as for routine inpatient care. Some of these infusions and procedures should relieve the overcrowded outpatient clinic. The nursing staff will be separate from the oncology inpatient unit, a 30-bed full-service unit.

A major research component of this unit will be to see if we can improve the quality of palliative care by concentrating it in the hands of those who prefer to provide it, and reduce unnecessary use, cost, and inconsistency in care. Patients will be admitted to the unit from both medicine and surgical units. Most patients are expected to be indigent people who have no other alternatives, but the unit will welcome everyone. We will also accept patients coming from the outpatient clinic or their homes for standard admissions, and will provide a respite to patients' family caregivers. A "pre/post comparison" will be made, using the Massey Cancer Center's database, to compare MCV-VCU patients treated in the previous two years to the first 100 patients treated in the palliative care unit. People will be matched for illness, demographic characteristics, and length of survival. Multivariate regression analysis will be done to learn what characteristics predict lower resource use and lower total inpatient care.

Our hypothesis is that total resource use and the cost of daily inpatient care can be reduced by increasing the volume of patients per practitioner. In nearly all other specialties studied, high clinical volume has been associated with better quality of care, and in some instances with better quality and lower cost (Hillner and Smith, 1998; Hillner, Smith, and Desch, 2000). For example, the death rate for esophagectomy is 14 percent at low-volume hospitals but only to 3 percent at high-volume hospitals. The survival rate for breast cancer patients treated by specialized centers or high-volume surgeons is better by 5 to 8 percent per 100 women at five years than the rate after low-volume care. The relative risk of death from breast cancer is 1.6 percent at low-volume New York hospitals compared to high-volume ones (Begg et al., 1998; Gillis and Hole, 1996; Sainsbury et al., 1995; Roohan et al., 1998). Costs can routinely be reduced by 10–15 percent by standardizing surgical care with clinical practice guidelines for breast, lung, gynecologic, and genitourinary patients (Katterhagen, 1996; Patton and Katterhagen, 1994; Morris et al., 1997; Litwin et al., 1996; Litwin et al., 1997). There are no comparable data for palliative care patients, although data do show that the use of a care coordinator can preserve the quality of care and reduce its costs by 40 percent (Rafferty et al., 1996; Addington-Hall et al., 1992; Institute of Medicine/National Academy of Sciences, 2000).

A strategic alliance to improve regional palliative care began in 1997 with discussions between Sister Joanne Lappetito, vice president in charge of mission for the Bon Secours Regional Health Care Program, and MCV-VCU. Bon Secours operates an outpatient hospice in the Richmond area with a typical census of 50–100 patients. It is a not-for-profit organization that shared the goals of MCV-VCU in providing care regardless of payment and seemed very compatible. MCV-VCU did not want to duplicate services by opening a

separate hospice. (Hospice services are underused in central Virginia. In 1996 the Connecticut Hospice, under contract to Thomas Hospice, estimated that only about 20 percent of the outpatient hospice needs were being met in the Richmond area.) We began a series of meetings with administration officials from both sides to merge the two institutions' outpatient hospices. However, this project was unsuccessful. The volume of indigent care at MCV-VCU—60 percent of the indigent care in the state, nearly 100 percent in the city—was daunting to Bon Secours. Unlike MCV-VCU, Bon Secours would get no payment from the state for such care. There was also speculation that a merger might shift charitable donations from one institution to another. No formal alliance occurred.

With so much indigent care, and so many insured patients preferring suburban hospitals with better parking, we have been struggling financially and are in danger of becoming an inner-city hospital like Chicago's Cook County. We have two separate types of practice, although we try to provide one level of care. We perform nearly all the chemotherapy and radiation for indigent patients in central Virginia because those procedures are expensive and because poor people have historically come to MCV-VCU. Medicaid in Virginia is among the most restrictive in the United States. The three teaching institutions in Virginia do receive some state funds as partial compensation for indigent care. These patients are treated in the hospitals' indigent-care clinics, often at different places or times from "private practice" patients of the same doctors and nurses. Until 2000, the physicians received little or no compensation for seeing these patients. It is a tribute to the MCV-VCU system that all patients receive the same care even so. What differs is that patients in the indigent-care clinics are typically seen by house officers or fellows under direct faculty supervision.

We have contracted with Bon Secours and the other local hospices, both for-profit and not-for-profit, to hospitalize their patients when they need inpatient care. This contract has been standardized. Approximately 90 percent of the per diem fees stay with the MCV-VCU Hospital, and about 10 percent are returned to the outpatient hospice for administration. We hope this improves the hospices' income, as a major problem for our patients had been lack of continuity after we discharged them. The unofficial alliance represents many lost opportunities for MCV-VCU. We lost the chances for high volume and good outcomes at lower cost and for efficiencies of scale and combined marketing programs. The loose affiliation may not produce any strong working relationships or team building. The use of many separate outpatient hospices increases the likelihood

of poor communication and impedes standardization. It also speaks loudly about competition among not-for-profits and about all institutions' fear of providing too much indigent care, even when that is an organization's mission.

Inspiration and Motivation of Thomas J. Smith

Compassionate care of both the living and the dying has been a theme in my medical training, and my personal characteristics and medical mentors have influenced it. Before entering medicine, I was shaped by the ethic of personal service and compassion found in Quaker meetings of the Society of Friends, and exposure to those involved in community service has been central to my life for about 40 years.

During medical education at Yale from 1974 to 1979, no one was specifically interested in hospice or palliative care. The best generalist physicians—long before the idea of a subspecialty in general internal medicine—were hematologists and oncologists. Without any particular fanfare, they saw curative and noncurative care as an integral part of what physicians did. Helping a dying faculty member to plan an endowed lectureship for women in medicine in her name convinced me that advance planning at the end of life is important.

My residency at the University of Pennsylvania was typical training in internal medicine, with no focus on palliative care. The university did not have a palliative care program, although Dr. Michael Levy, then a Penn fellow, eventually became a national expert in the area. Fellowship training in hematology/oncology at the Medical College of Virginia and in the National Cancer Institute's Biological Response Modifiers Program convinced me that compassionate care of both the living and the dying was important but not a special focus. No one during my fellowship training had a specific interest in palliative care, although the best "treating" doctor provided excellent pain relief. Once again, this was just something that good doctors did.

Several mentors have helped guide my work in this field. The first is Patrick J. Coyne, R.N., M.S., who has become a national expert in palliative care. We began working together in 1993–1994, when he planned a trip to Tanzania with the American Medical Team for Africa and dragged me along as an experienced oncologist. During our three weeks in East Africa and in subsequent discussions, we began thinking about a palliative care program for MCV-VCU. Another role model, although not a mentor, is Dr. David Weissman, whom I first met through the American Association for Cancer Education.

As early as 1990, he was promulgating the idea that cancer doctors were obligated to provide better treatment at the end of life. The "lunatic fringe" in the American Society of Clinical Oncology kept pushing the idea that palliation was an essential part of care. Other role models included Dr. Kathleen Foley for writing and lecturing on team management, Dr. June Dahl for her work in establishing the State Cancer Pain Initiatives, and Michael Levy for continuing to write that oncology training should include palliative care.

The idea of creating a palliative care program at MCV-VCU arose from discussions during 1993–94. A critical mass of people interested in it was slowly developing, including Pat Coyne, Dr. James Shaw, a few others, and me. The chief nursing administrator for the hospital was keenly interested in developing such a program, having worked in palliative care for nearly 20 years. Funding through the Project on Death in America was instrumental in making this program happen. The PDIA let us focus on end-of-life care and provided recognition from the outside world that this was a significant service that our hospital group should provide. The decision to develop the program was not specifically inspired by any other program or another colleague's efforts or by a particular patient or group of patients. It grew because Pat

Coyne and I thought it was important. We combed the literature for other palliative care programs in big hospitals with a large, urban, poor population. We found none.

Our success in creating the Rural Cancer Outreach Program, with its concentration on both curative and palliative care, influenced our decision to pursue the idea of creating a palliative care program. Dr. Chris Desch, nurses Nancy Kane and Cyndy Simonson, and I began the Rural Cancer Outreach Program in 1989. Under the outreach program, rural and academic health centers have a team of oncologists and oncology nurse clinical specialists who travel to rural hospitals several times a month to provide comprehensive cancer treatment, including palliative care. The rural hospitals have several oncology nurses who live in the community and a small cadre of physicians interested in cancer care, including palliative care. This program has been highly successful in bringing state-of-the-art care to both prosperous and medically underserved people in rural areas. It has generated substantial profit for the rural hospitals by keeping the care in the area; has reduced the overall cost of care and the cost of admissions from rural areas to MCV-VCU Hospital by about 40 percent; and has improved the quality of care (Desch et al., 1992; Desch et al., 1999; Smith et al., 1996). When we started this program, rural hospitals used virtually no morphine, and minuscule amounts of any pain reliever except Demerol. As we have said in other publications, we emphasized that cancer patients are entitled to pain and symptom management, whether being treated with curative or palliative intent. We have seen dramatic increases in the amount of analgesics used at rural hospitals. This program's success told us that at least some parts of medical treatment could be improved.

Nurses and physicians in our department have welcomed our work in palliative care. That may be because we keep palliative care within the mainstream of cancer treatment. It may be because we succeed in what we do, are competent in other areas, and have a national reputation, too. *Or it may be because we are pushy*. We have always approached palliative care as an integral part of oncology practice. In general, the colleagues who are least interested in comprehensive palliative care are the most interested in turning over end-of-life care to those of us who *are* interested. This may be specific to our institution. We have too many patients, and patients are sometimes seen as a liability, not an asset.

Money may not be the only currency at academic institutions, but it certainly gets attention. The institution did not pay much attention to our efforts until we received funding from the Project on Death in America and subsequent funding from the Jessie Ball DuPont Fund and the Thomas

Hospice Foundation. This high visibility, combined with high-visibility initiatives through the AMA, American Society of Clinical Oncology, Oncology Nursing Society, and others, gave us a stamp of social approval.

My personal attitude toward palliative care has not changed much since the early days of the program. The main frustrations are these: (1) the inability to cure more patients; (2) the inability to relieve symptoms completely in a small number of patients; (3) the lack of universal health care, so that indigent care becomes concentrated at one place; (4) the undervaluing of palliative care by insurers; and (5) the persistently unrealistic expectations of some patients and families. This last frustration is reaching epidemic proportions. It is increasingly difficult to convince patients that we have no good anticancer treatment for some of them, and they sometimes bring me 200 protocols to examine. I am less patient with this than I used to be, and I have less time for it.

The structure of oncology reimbursement deserves special mention and explanation. About 50–66 percent of most oncologists' practice comes from buying and selling chemotherapy drugs unrelated to evaluation and management (Kurowski, 1998; Smyth, 1993). This arrangement compensates oncologists for the expense of the drugs, makes sure the drugs are available, and raises overall compensation to allow for the intense, time-consuming nature of oncology. Most academic institutions give this income to the hospital. That means that I will always make one-third of what my colleagues in practice do, even for the same work. Within this system, chemotherapy administration is rewarded most. Sixty-eight percent of my reimbursable charges come from administering chemotherapy (J-codes) and not from evaluating and managing patients. Whether current compensation represents a conflict of interest or changes practice patterns is not known for certain, although we do know that private-practice oncologists use much more expensive colony stimulating factors than academic or staff doctors in HMOs (Bennett et al., 1996; Bennett et al., 1999). I do know that if I stopped giving chemotherapy and moved to a practice based on counseling without infusions, my income would drop by two-thirds. We have attempted to modify this effect by careful attention to every billing detail and by maximizing reimbursement on all services we do provide. As long as payment exists for expensive radiation, such as erythropoietin, pamidronate, and radiation pharmaceuticals, then the incentives of chemotherapy can be applied to palliative interventions. We worry that a switch to capitated payments would send us back to using only morphine suppositories.

The most rewarding and meaningful aspect of cancer care is the appreciation of patients and their family members for good and reasonable care. Again, we make little distinction between symptom relief in treatment for testicular cancer and symptom relief and palliation for those at the end of life. Exploration of spiritual and existential issues can be just as profound during both phases of an illness, too. I differ from many of my colleagues in that I persist in providing curative treatment and palliative chemotherapy as well as other types of palliative care. This is my personal choice, but I believe that most cancer doctors should consider it.

 Program Development
. . . .

The initial goals of the MCV-VCU program were to create a geographically separate inpatient unit that could be used for clinical practice, research, education, and even fund raising. We feared that beds dispersed throughout the hospital would not provide an appropriate focus for any of those goals. The goals have evolved over time, influenced by the failure of the palliative care unit at another local hospital due to poor location and poor understanding of the needs of patients and physicians. Understanding of current referral patterns is probably more important than major attempts to change them. *We have learned to put an inpatient unit where people will want to go, make it*

geographically and physically attractive, and not try to force major changes in physicians' referral patterns.

The second goal in developing our program was to make a not-for-profit alliance between health care programs providing palliative care. We did this to prevent duplication of services, concentrate per diem payments in one outpatient hospice at Bon Secours, expand their volume substantially to obtain economies of scale, and promote cooperation between the two institutions. The failure of this program, except on an informal basis, has been sobering. The ability of a for-profit local hospice to work with us has been heartening, suggesting that for-profit and not-for-profit status are less important than being willing to assume a small financial risk for a large financial gain in the future.

The key steps in the initial program development were gathering a critical mass of people with a like interest, specifically Pat Coyne, Cyndy Simonson, James Shaw, and me, among others and then, *persistence, persistence, persistence.* The concentration on palliative care in the Rural Cancer Outreach Program showed us that palliative care could be used throughout hospital systems. The other key steps were the involvement of the hospital's administrative decision makers from the beginning and our openly sharing with them the risks and benefits of setting up a program. This program will never be a major revenue source for the medical center. However, it can provide state-of-the-art care as part of the mission of the NCI-sponsored cancer center—teaching, research, and service. Grants from the Jessie Ball DuPont Fund and the Project on Death in America were also useful. They made the administration sit up and take notice, and nearly $300,000 sitting unused in the bank is a strong incentive to force the space for a unit. The persistence of Pat Coyne and others in steadfastly pushing the program at every opportunity has been crucial.

We have come across many barriers in putting this program into place, especially administrative, bureaucratic, and financial barriers. *The lack of financial forecasting for such units has been a big handicap. We could not show that such a unit either broke even or saved money at any other U.S. institution.* This program represents a substantial new effort and has required time, planning, and fortitude; all are scarce at beleaguered urban institutions. The reluctance to see this program as essential could be construed as either shortsighted or wise. Wearing my administrator's hat, I myself see such programs as a major risk. They displace existing programs, require short-term renovation costs and continuing personnel costs, and invite concern about lost long-term opportunities: What if we had put a profitable cardiac cath unit into the same space or a chemo infusion center? (Smith, 1993).

Personnel and staff recruitment has been another formidable barrier. Those of us interested in the program have other substantial responsibilities. It has been hard to free time and energy without clear-cut funding to pay salaries—other than potential patient revenue or, even worse, just the possibility of smaller losses. The lack of an academic focus has been another barrier to recruitment. We academics are evaluated by one form of productivity or another, like grants, clinical dollars, or publications. We have not been able to point to other programs that have succeeded by any of these standards. This is especially troubling to junior colleagues who have no established track records in other areas. They ask themselves, "Why take a chance on this? Why not go into private practice and make a lot more money without the hassles or do other types of clinical research?" We have a core of good people here, but our situation will always be tenuous in an academic setting unless we can come up with publishable research or an honest-to-goodness clinical educator track.

To diminish these barriers, we have used persistence, persistence, and persistence, as already noted. We continually stress that palliative care is "the right thing to do" even if it does not make a lot of money. Both Pat Coyne and I have the advantage of having reasonably successful careers in other areas so that this "side job" is not the center of our work. We have stressed to hospital administration that this program can be a source of substantial revenue in the future, and that it can let us test the reasonable hypothesis that concentrating end-of-life care in the hands of those who like to do it will save money in the long run.

We have not been in operation long enough to assure that the program will remain faithful to its original mission. Personnel continuity will be critical to that. Both Pat Coyne and I have made long-term commitments to the program, like most of the others involved in it. We want this to work for the sake of the community.

We have tried to forecast the financial viability of the program. Financial analysis of the Rural Outreach Program suggests that such forecasts can be made. We have argued all along that patients who need palliative care are already in the hospital and that a low-cost unit to care for them frees standard medical-surgical beds for other patients, therefore generating revenue. We have emphasized that the program will last only if it is financially viable and have taken steps to test that hypothesis. We have not been at work long enough to know whether the program will survive after its creators have

left. Our experience with the Rural Cancer Outreach Program suggests that a low-revenue, high-visibility program that is socially good will continue if personnel who share its goals are recruited.

If we were starting all over again, I would insist that all promises be made in writing with a time line attached. However, that would clash with the culture of our organization, and I doubt that this strategy would have worked. I would also have asked the other hospice programs right up front how much indigent care they were willing to consider. If the answer is only a few percent, then collaborations with such programs cannot work, given our high level of indigent care. From the hospice's perspective, though, why give a number? If it's 3 percent, that's already 2 percent higher than the other businesses in town. If it's 1 percent, they would be in trouble with the Certificate of Need regulators. And if they agree to 15 percent, their boards would have a conniption. After all, MCV-VCU gets money from the state to take care of poor people, so let *them* do it. (One not-for-profit religious-based health care system has now closed two downtown hospitals to transfer their beds to the affluent suburbs. Perhaps that is the wise long-term solution, but it isolates the urban poor at our center, and sets up this nonprofit to serve most of the insured suburbanites who might otherwise come to MCV-VCU.

Institutional Culture

The hospital culture that facilitated the development of the program includes its academic and service missions; its long commitment to serving all, including the poor; and its tradition of letting innovators develop new programs. There is a strong ethic here of taking care of everyone without regard to ability to pay, even providing high-dose chemotherapy and stem-cell transplants.

Two aspects of the hospital culture hindered the development of the program. One is appropriate conservatism regarding new programs that might present substantial financial or care burdens down the road. The other is the lack of centralized decision-making authority among the Hospital, University, Medical School, Cancer Center, Department of Internal Medicine, and University Physician Group. No one, or everyone, is in charge. *This is where entrepreneurship is critical!*

The most vital support came from Carl Fischer, the hospital's chief executive officer (whose wife is an oncology nurse), and later from Donna Katen-Bahensky, the chief operating officer. Essential support also came from Barbara Farley, the hospital's chief of nursing. We obtained their support by explaining the program to them several times, reminding them of it during lulls in

development, and obtaining grants to show external endorsement of the program. We gave regular updates to the dean of the medical school, the president of the university, and the heads of the various groups of physicians.

These efforts were only partly successful in getting the university to free space for the palliative care unit. The departments that were using that space vigorously resisted being moved and having to change their outpatient and inpatient programs. (If I had been in their shoes, I would have resisted in exactly the same way!) It has taken extreme persistence by a number of us, particularly the new chief operating officer hired expressly to take on difficult projects, to find alternative space for them. To get the space by the spring of 1999, we had to threaten to resign and start the program at a competing hospital across town.

We have not tried to increase the program's visibility and credibility in the hospital community at large. Word is already out "on the street" that the program is open, and we have more requests from medical students, interns, and residents to work on it than we can handle. We will provide the very best care possible, in a convenient and accessible setting, as well as the best teaching in the hospital. We have not existed long enough to contrast the program today with the program at its inception.

Specific thanks and credit must be given to the Thomas Hospice for joining forces with us. As noted above, Thomas was Richmond's first inpatient hospice, and was in existence from 1971 until 1995 when Columbia/HCA bought their hospital. Their negotiations with the Bon Secours program fell apart on issues of name and control. Thomas invited us to partner with them, completely out of the blue. Although they have not been able to solve our problems of diffused leadership and slow decision-making, they have been a persistent force in making the hospital find space. Development offices have recognized their potential as well. They can be a substantial help in fund raising, expand our community visibility, and help us reach a group of people whom we might not otherwise reach.

I. Institutional Information

    A. Name of hospital and program

        1. Thomas Hospice Palliative Care Unit at Medical College of Virginia Hospitals of Virginia Commonwealth University

        2. Informal Strategic Alliance of Palliative Care in Central Virginia

    B. Directors

        Thomas J. Smith, MD, Medical Director

        Patrick J. Coyne, RN, MS, Director of Nursing Services

        Laurel J. Lyckholm, MD, Director of Fellowship Program and Palliative Care Education

        Cynthia J. Simonson, RN, MS, Acting Director for Nursing for Massey Cancer Center

        Allison Larson, RN, MS, Nursing Manager

    C. Program start: May 2000

    D. Hospital setting: Urban

    E. Type of institution: Academic

        1. Affiliated medical school: Medical College of Virginia Campus of Virginia Commonwealth University

        2. Affiliated residency training program: Medical College of Virginia Campus of Virginia Commonwealth University, Department of Internal Medicine, Department of Radiation/Oncology, and Department of Surgery

    F. Number of beds in our system: 700

    G. Health Care System

        1. 1 hospital affiliate

        2. 1 long-term care affiliate

II. Program Characteristics

    A. Clinical Staff

        1. Physician specialties: medical oncology, surgical oncology

        2. Nurses' training: Specific interest in palliative care

        3. Social workers: One, to cover both inpatient oncology unit and palliative care unit

        4. Other health care providers: Chaplaincy program; nutrition and dietician programs shared with oncology; support group system shared with Massey Cancer Center; patient family education and library services shared with Massey Cancer Center; pediatrics as needed; geriatrics; hospitalists.

B. Research Staff

    1. Dedicated research staff: We have a 25 percent salary commitment for a programmer-analyst to make the pre- and post-comparisons already set up through the grant from the Jessie Ball DuPont Fund.

    2. Who they are: To be named. Similar research has been done by Drs. Tom Smith, Bruce Hillner, Lynne Penberthy, and others through the outcomes research program of the Massey Cancer Center.

PERSONNEL

Physician medical director

Nurse manager

Clinical nurse: 9 FTE (full-time equivalent)

Licensed practical nurse: 1.5 FTE

Patient care technician: 4.5 FTE

Office specialist: .7 FTE

Volunteer coordinator: .5 FTE

Registered nurse: .5 FTE

C. Administrative Staff

    1. Medical director

    2. Nursing director

    3. Nursing program coordinator

    4. Volunteer coordinator

    5. Development officer assigned to the project through the consortium of the Medical College and the Hospital

D. Clinical Characteristics

    1. Hospital department or division: Medical/Surgical Nursing

    2. Consult Service: The consult service, established many years ago, will be restarted October 2000 with the addition of Dr. Kirk Payne.

    3. Dedicated inpatient palliative care unit: 11 beds

    4. Dedicated inpatient hospice unit: Same as above

    5. Home hospice program: No specific program. There is a large program, MCV-VCU Care at Home. For many years, a home visitation program has been run

through the Division of General Internal Medicine home care program and the MCV-VCU geriatrics program. We will collaborate with several local hospices.

E. Patient Population

   1. Number per month on the inpatient unit: Anticipate 8–11 beds

   2. Number per month on the consult service: Anticipate 20 (October 2000)

   3. Number per month receiving home-care: To be determined (TBD)

   4. Number per month in hospice: TBD

   5. Average length of stay on the program

      a. Inpatient: TBD

      b. Outpatient: TBD

   6. Demographics of patient population (diagnosis, age, ethnicity, etc.): TBD; anticipate 100% adults, 20% or more indigent, 50% African American

F. Estimated funding sources

   1. Foundation grants: 10%

   2. Federal grants: None

   3. Endowments: 5%

   4. Charity: 5%

   5. Hospital support: 10%

   6. Medical school support: None

   7. Clinical income: 70%

   8. Other sources: None

G. Educational Component

   1. Programmatic types: TBD

   2. Trainees

      a. Fellows: 1 per month, elective

      b. Residents: 1 per month, elective

      c. Medical Students: 1 per month, elective

      d. Faculty/Colleagues: 0

      e. Nurses: TBD

      f. Social Workers: interns

      g. Public: 0

III. Research Component: Funding Sources

    A.   Federal grants: none

    B.   Foundation Grants: 100% (see box)

    C.   Industry: TBD

    D.   Intramural: none

GRANTS

Medtronics, Inc. Minneapolis, Minn., 1999.

Randomized clinical trial to evaluate the efficacy, cost-effectiveness, and impact on quality of life of implantable narcotic delivery systems vs. comprehensive medical management. $2.5 million

Hunton Foundation, Richmond, Virginia, 1999

Creation of an Education Center for hospice. $ 7,000

Jessie Ball DuPont Fund, Jacksonville, Florida, 1998–2001

Creation of a Palliative Care Unit to serve the medically underserved. $287,000/3 years

---

Thomas Hospice Palliative Care Unit at MCV-VCU

Projected Funding Sources

Clinical Income	70%	■
Foundation Grants	10%	
Hospital Support	10%	■
Charity	5%	■
Endowments	3%	■

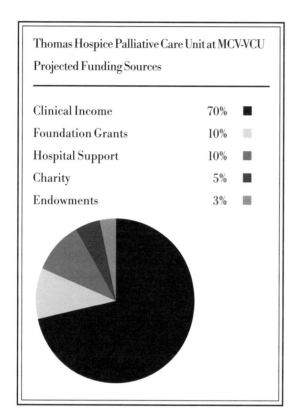

Thomas Hospice Palliative Care Unit at MCV-VCU

Projected Payer Sources

Medicare	40%	■
Medicaid	20%	
Insurance	20%	■
Indigent	20%	■

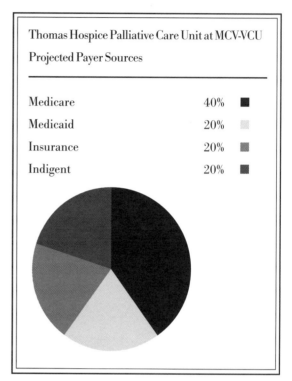

REFERENCES

Addington-Hall, J.M., L.D. MacDonald, H.R. Anderson, et al. 1992. Randomized Controlled Trial of Effects of Coordinating Care for Terminally Ill Cancer Patients. *British Medical Journal*, 305:1317–22.

Begg, C.B., L. Cramer, W. Hoskins, and M. Brennan. 1998. Impact of Hospital Volume on Operative Mortality for Major Cancer Surgery. *Journal of the American Medical Association*, 280:1747–51.

Bennett, C., T. Smith, J. Weeks, et al. 1996. Use of Hematopoietic Colony Stimulating Factors: The American Society of Clinical Oncology. *Journal of Clinical Oncology*, 14:2511–20.

Bennett, C.L., J. Weeks, M.R. Somerfield, J. Feinglass, and T.J. Smith. 1999. Use of Hematopoietic Colony Stimulating Factors: Comparison of the 1994 and 1997 American Society of Clinical Oncology Surveys Regarding ASCO Clinical Practice Guidelines. *Journal of Clinical Oncology*, 17:3676–81.

Desch, C.E., K. Grasso, M. McCue, D. Buonaiuto, M.K. Johantgen, et al. 1999. A Rural Cancer Outreach Program Lowers Patient Care Costs and Benefits Both the Rural Hospitals and Sponsoring Academic Medical Center. *The Journal of Rural Health*, 15(2):157–67.

Desch, C.E., T.J. Smith, C.A. Briendel, C.J. Simonson, and N. Kane. 1992. Cancer Treatment in Rural Areas. *Hospital and Health Services Administration*, 37:449–63.

Gillis, C.R., and D.J. Hole. 1996. Survival Outcome of Care by Specialist Surgeons in Breast Cancer: A Study of 3,786 Patients in the West of Scotland. *British Medical Journal*, 312:145–48.

Hillner, B.E., and T.J. Smith. 1998. Hospital Volume and Patient Outcomes in Major Cancer Surgery: A Catalyst for Quality Assessment and Concentration of Cancer Services. *Journal of the American Medical Association*, 280:1783–4.

Hillner, B.E., T.J. Smith, and C.E. Desch. 2000. Hospital and Physician Volume or Specialization and Outcomes in Cancer Treatment: Importance in Quality of Cancer Care. *Journal of Clinical Oncology*, 18(11):2327–40.

Institute of Medicine/National Academy of Science. 2000. *Ensuring Quality Cancer Care.* Washington, D.C.

Katterhagen, G. 1996. Physician Compliance with Outcome-Based Guidelines and Clinical Pathways in Oncology. *Oncology,* November, 113–21.

Kurowski, B. 1998. Six Key Challenges in Oncology Disease Management. *Disease Management,* 1:99–105.

Litwin, M.S., R.B. Smith, A. Thind, N. Reccius, M. Blanco-Yarosh, and J.B. deKernion. 1996. Cost-Efficient Radical Prostatectomy with a Clinical Care Path. *Journal of Urology,* 155:989–93.

Litwin, M.S., A.I. Shpall, and F. Dorey. 1997. Patient Satisfaction with Short Stays for Radical Prostatectomy. *Urology,* 49(6): 898–906.

Morris, M., C. Levenback, T.W. Burke, Y. Dejesus, K.R. Lucas, and D.M. Gershenson. 1997. An Outcomes Management Program in Gynecological Oncology. *Obstetrics and Gynecology,* 89(4):485–92.

Patton, M.D., and J.G. Katterhagen. 1994. Critical Pathways in Oncology: Aligning Resource Expenditures with Clinical Outcomes. *Journal of Oncology Management,* July/August:16–21.

Rafferty, J.P., J.M. Addington-Hall, L.D. MacDonald, et al. 1996. A Randomized Controlled Trial of the Cost-Effectiveness of a District Co-ordinating Service for Terminally Ill Cancer Patients. *Palliative Medicine,* 10:151–61.

Roohan, P., N. Bickell, M. Baptiste, G. Therriault, E. Ferrara, and A.L. Siu. 1998. Hospital Volume Differences and Five-Year Survival from Breast Cancer. *American Jornal of Public Health,* 88:454–7.

Sainsbury, R., R. Haward, L. Rider, C. Johnstone, and C. Round. 1995. Influence of Clinician Workload and Patterns of Treatment on Survival from Breast Cancer. *Lancet,* 345:1265–70.

Smith, T.J. 1993. Which Hat Do I Wear? *Journal of the American Medical Association,* 270:1657–9.

Smith, T.J., C.E. Desch, C.J. Simonson, and N.E. Kane. 1991. Teaching Subspecialty Cancer Medicine in Rural Hospitals. The Cancer Outreach Program as a Model. *Journal of Cancer Education,* 6:235–40.

Smith, T.J., C.E. Desch, M.A. Grasso, et al. 1996. The Rural Cancer Outreach Program: Clinical and Financial Analysis of Palliative and Curative Care for an Underserved Population. *Cancer Treatment Review,* 22:97–101.

Smyth, A. 1993. Reimbursement Issues for the Oncologist. *Oncology Reimbursement,* 1:1–4.

Pain and Palliative Care Service
Memorial Sloan-Kettering Cancer Center

Richard Payne and Kathleen M. Foley

Inspiration and Motivation

Pain management and research has been a focus at Memorial Sloan-Kettering Cancer Center since the 1940s, as a result of the pioneering work of Dr. Raymond Houde and staff members in defining analgesic potencies (Houde, Wallenstein and Rogers, 1960). A comprehensive Pain and Palliative Care Program began in 1975 when Dr. Kathleen M. Foley joined the Department of Neurology. Before the program expanded to include palliative care, it was called the Pain Service. Dr. Foley worked to understand the epidemiology and demography of cancer pain and to develop assessments, treatments, and research and training focusing on cancer pain from a neurological perspective. At the time, the common view was that pain was a neurological complication of cancer; it was the most common reason why patients with neurological disease and cancer turned to their physicians. At the outset, Dr. Foley recognized that patients with cancer-related pain needed not only expert assessment and management of neurological disorders and pain but an emphasis on improving function and overall quality of life.

The Pain and Palliative Care Service at Memorial Sloan-Kettering Cancer Center (MSKCC) has a long history. Its excellent training and education have affected at least three other major pain and palliative care programs in the United States. For 25 years, the single most important force in this history has been the personal commitment and superb leadership of Dr. Kathleen Foley, who has devoted her career to this effort.

In the mid-1970s, Dr. Foley began seeing patients in the outpatient medical clinic with Dr. Houde, in the analgesic studies section of the Department of Medicine. With the help of Dr. Houde and Ada Rogers, R.N., Dr. Foley developed an inpatient pain consultation service in the Department of Neurology. Robert F. Kaiko, Ph.D., a pharmacologist, joined the group, and a series of studies of the epidemiology and demography of cancer pain was undertaken. The group also conducted pharmaceutical-based studies (Foley, 1979; Foley et al., 1978; Kaiko et al., 1978).

In 1978, the Department of Neurology designated funds to support a fellow, and a training program began. From 1978 to 1986 it was supported predominantly by philanthropy. These funds paid the salary of one to three fellows a year, who were typically neurologists, and who gained experience and expertise in both neuro-oncology and pain. The pain fellows attended the outpatient pain clinic one day a week, provided inpatient consultations, and attended weekly teaching rounds and conferences. Dr. Richard Payne, who began training in the New York Hospital–Cornell University Medical Center neurology residency program in 1979, learned of the teaching of Drs. Foley and Houde and Ada Rogers, R.N., and the work of the Pain Service through required clinical rotations at Memorial Sloan-Kettering Cancer Center.

The Department of Neurology at MSKCC established two training tracks. Neurologists who had completed residency training could continue their preparation as neuro-oncology fellows or as pain fellows. Both fellowship tracks required a two-year commitment. The neuro-oncology fellows did a three-month rotation on the Pain Service. Like the pain fellows, they were under the primary supervision of Dr. Foley. This experience provided them with expertise in pain management and palliative care. The Pain Service fellowship was originally integrated with the Anesthesiology Department and allowed anesthesiologists to do a one-month rotation with the Pain Service. The integration ended in 1997 because both programs grew, and anesthesiology trainees needed to fulfill additional certification requirements that were unavailable to neurologists.

During this period, Dr. Foley received a grant from the Dupont Pharmaceutical Company to support an observership program for health care professionals interested in pain and palliative care. Approximately 40 to 60 people a year have come from all over the world to participate in this program since its inception. Observers spent weeks or months with the Pain Service learning enough about cancer pain management to develop similar programs at their own institutions.

In 1979, Dr. Foley began working with Dr. Charles Inturrisi, associate professor of pharmacology at Cornell University Medical College. Dr. Inturrisi was instrumental in developing the research program of the Pain Service and has collaborated on many pharmaceutical studies and grants. Dr. Inturrisi has also contributed greatly to the development of the clinical research training program and has served as mentor for many pain fellows who eventually became leaders of other programs, including Dr. Payne. In 1979, Dr. Foley received the first of a series of NIH grants supported by the National Cancer Institute to examine the pharmacokinetics and pharmacodynamics of opioid analgesics. This endeavor expanded into 16 years of NIH research funding and multiple studies funded by the pharmaceutical industry, with the collaboration of Drs. Houde and Inturrisi.

In 1981, the clinical pain service based in the Department of Neurology and the research program based in the analgesic studies section of the Department of Medicine merged into the Pain Service in the Department of Neurology. Dr. Foley was named chief of the Pain Service. The Pain Service was then composed of Dr. Foley, Dr. Gavril Pasternak, Dr. Raymond

Houde, Mr. Stanley Wallenstein, Dr. Robert F. Kaiko, Ms. Ada Rogers, three to five analgesic nurse observers, a data manager, and one or two clinical pain fellows. The Departments of Neurology and Medicine provided Dr. Foley and Dr. Houde with space and clinical and administrative support; their salaries were funded by research grants and direct patient care. Most other members of the Pain Service were paid from philanthropic funds or pharmaceutical funds for individual studies.

In the early 1980s, Dr. Foley and a committee of patients' families and friends developed the Hemingway Fund for Pain Research and Education. The committee's goal was to raise money for Dr. Foley's work in educating and training future physicians and nurses in pain management and research. The Hemingway Fund has been the primary philanthropy supporting the Pain Service for nearly 20 years.

In 1981, we developed the Supportive Care Program for cancer patients at home. Nurses provided continuity of care and 24-hour supervision for dying patients with significant pain and palliative care needs (Coyle, 1989). Dr. Kathleen Foley serves as the program's medical director and Nessa Coyle, A.N.P., as its nurse director. Additional staff members have included a psychiatrist, a social worker and, for a brief period of time, a music therapist. The Supportive Care Program was funded for its

first four years by philanthropic funds, which paid the salaries of two full-time clinical nurse specialists and a social worker. Shortly thereafter, we created the Supportive Care Program Philanthropic Fund to meet nonreimbursed patient care needs; it also provided additional money to train physicians and nurses. The importance of the Supportive Care Program was recognized by the hospital administration, which assumed its funding in 1985. This reliable funding for nonreimbursable patient care needs is critical to the success of the Pain and Palliative Care Program.

The Supportive Care Program remains an essential part of the Pain and Palliative Care Service to this day. Patients enter the program when they require close supervision and coordination of services within the community. Nurses in the Supportive Care Program work as a team with physicians in the Pain and Palliative Care Service to provide telephone advice, write prescriptions, and make house calls (Coyle, 1995).

In 1982, after a year as chief resident in neurology at New York Hospital–Cornell Medical Center, Dr. Richard Payne began a two-year clinical and research fellowship with Drs. Kathleen Foley and Charles Inturrisi. Dr. Payne was attracted to the program through his clinical exposure to the service as a neurology resident, and Dr. Foley, an attending physician in Neurology, had become his mentor before he began his fellowship. As a neurology resident at Memorial Sloan-Kettering, Dr. Payne saw several young patients who were physically and emotionally devastated by cancer metastasis, neurological impairments, and pain. He was impressed by the professional expertise of Dr. Foley and the interdisciplinary team on the Pain Service as they supervised his clinical training. Dr. Foley's example as a role model and her early mentoring were critical in his career development. They are the reason he entered the field.

Dr. Payne's early research as a pain fellow, funded by a clinical scholar's grant through the Sloan-Kettering Institute, involved the development of an animal model to evaluate pharmacokinetic-pharmacodynamic relationships of opioids administered by the spinal route (Payne, Madson, Harvey, et al., 1986). He conducted the research at Cornell University Medical College under the supervision of Dr. Charles Inturrisi, professor of pharmacology and adjunct member of the Sloan-Kettering Institute. The cross affiliations of researchers and mentors in the Cornell-Memorial Sloan-Kettering Cancer Center complex were instrumental in Dr. Payne's career development.

After completing his fellowship in 1984, Dr. Payne joined Drs. Foley, Houde, and Pasternak as the fourth faculty member of the Pain Service in the Department of Neurology. Dr. Payne's qualifications for a faculty position were significantly enhanced by his successful application to the Robert Wood Johnson Minority Faculty Development Program. He was part of the first cohort of physician-scientists chosen for these awards, which provided partial salary support and research funding to pursue his studies in opioid pharmacology; Dr. Inturrisi at Cornell Medical College and Dr. Foley served as faculty mentors for the award. Dr. Payne remained on the faculty at MSKCC until 1987, then left to develop a program of pain research and management at the University of Cincinnati–Veterans Administration Medical Center. In 1992, he went to lead the Pain and Symptom Management Program at the M. D. Anderson Cancer Center of the University of Texas. In 1998, Dr. Payne returned to MSKCC.

Pain and Palliative Care Programs at MSKCC in the 1990s

The 1990s saw continued growth, productivity, and prestige for the Pain Service at MSKCC. In 1987, after Dr. Payne left, Dr. Russell K. Portenoy joined the Service as an associate attending neurologist and director of analgesic studies. He served as principal investigator on many pharmaceutical studies and led the development of the Memorial Symptom Assessment Scale (MSAS), which has been validated and used internationally (Portenoy et al., 1994). Dr. Portenoy provided important research and clinical leadership and continued the long tradition of analgesic studies at MSKCC.

In 1996, the name of the Pain Service was changed to the Pain and Palliative Care Service, and Dr. Kathleen M. Foley and Dr. Russell K. Portenoy served as its co-chiefs. This name change recognized that the Pain Service had broadened its mission to encompass expertise in assessing and treating many additional physical symptoms, including fatigue, depression and psychological distress, dyspnea, etc. Furthermore, to assess and treat symptoms caused by intensive cancer treatment and by metastatic cancer required attention to medical, spiritual, and other aspects of palliative care at the end of life. Dr. Portenoy was expected to direct this initiative, allowing Dr. Foley to focus on World Health Organization programs in pain and palliative care.

Dr. Foley's creation and direction of a new funding agency, the Project on Death in America, in the mid-1990s significantly enhanced opportunities to advance the field of palliative and end-of-life care, and to reach the public at large. Her work there increased the emphasis on improved care of dying patients at MSKCC. Drs. Portenoy and Foley, in collaboration with the Nursing Department and nurses on the Pain and Palliative Care Service, initially led these efforts. As a result of these activities, we standardized nursing assessments and care of all patients dying within MSKCC. Collaboration expanded to the Department of Psychiatry in the areas of symptom assessment—like pain, fatigue, and depression—in patients with AIDS, and in the establishment of a program of bereavement services (Rosenfeld et al., 1999; Breitbart et al., 1998). These activities continue today.

In 1997, Dr. Portenoy left MSKCC to chair the Department of Pain Medicine and Palliative Care at Beth Israel Medical Center and become professor of neurology at Albert Einstein College of Medicine in New York. His departure provided an opportunity for Dr. Payne to return to MSKCC in 1998 as chief of the Pain and Palliative Care Service.

MSKCC's renewed commitment to research, education, and patient care in the Pain and Palliative Care Service made Dr. Payne's return as chief possible. Tangible evidence of this commitment includes the funding of a professorial chair for Dr. Payne; the allocation of institutional resources and fund-raising to establish a six-bed inpatient palliative care unit; full institutional support for 5.5 full-time Pain and Palliative Care faculty positions; partial fellowship support to expand the program to five positions; and additional space and other resources to expand clinical service and research. Most recently, the Service has established an endowed program to increase professional and patient education in pain management and palliative care.

In summary, the MSKCC Pain and Palliative Care Service has evolved over the past 25 years from a program based on the neurological study of pain to a program recognizing the broader implications of how cancer patients experience pain. Throughout its evolution, the program has continued a tradition of excellence and leadership in pain and palliative care research and patient care. Many individuals in the program have made major scientific contribution in the field. Drs. Foley, Pasternak, Inturrisi, and Portenoy are among the 20 most-cited authors in the pain and analgesia literature of the past 20 years (Fishman, et al., 1987; Foley and Inturrisi, 1986; Foley, Ventafridda, and Bonica, 1990; Kuhar and Pasternak, 1983; Payne, Patt, and Hill, 1998; Strassels et al., 1999; and WHO, 1986, 1990, and 1998). They and Dr. Payne have served as leaders in national professional and governmental organizations, such as the American Pain Society, American Academy of Pain Medicine, American Academy of Palliative and Hospice Medicine, National Institutes of Health, Agency for Health Care Policy and Research, and the Institute of Medicine, which have set policy and guidelines during the last 20 years. Faculty members and past trainees of the MSKCC program currently

edit major journals and textbooks in the field. Former trainees now lead, or are major contributors to, pain and palliative care programs in academic institutions in the United States, Canada, Italy, Israel, and Australia. Nursing leadership at the national and international level has been consistently excellent since 1975, as measured by contributions to the education of nurses and physicians, by editorship of major textbooks, and by numerous publications. This program has been a beacon in the field.

Departmental and Institutional Support

Dr. Jerome B. Posner, founding chair of the Neurology Department, was a critical influence in the initial recruitment of Dr. Foley and in the subsequent design and development of an independent service. Dr. Posner's consistent support permitted the development of the Service's clinical, research, and educational programs. The MSKCC Neurology Department provided seed money for the Service's infrastructure and fellows when no funds were available from other sources. In 1990, Dr. Posner facilitated the creation of an endowed chair for Dr. Foley in cancer pain research and education, which was funded specifically for Dr. Foley by the Society of Memorial Sloan-Kettering Cancer Center. Dr. Posner also played a key role in attracting Dr. Payne to the neurology residency program at Cornell and has consistently supported his career.

Dr. Paul Marks, president and CEO of MSKCC, and the various physicians-in-chief have consistently supported the Pain and Palliative Care Service. They have promoted its activities by focusing the institution's public relations and fundraising campaigns on the importance of managing pain for these patients and have sought media attention to the issue. Dr. Payne's return to MSKCC was possible because Dr. Marks committed considerable fundraising efforts and other resources to expanded pain and palliative care activities. Under his leadership, MSKCC raised $1 million during 1998 and 1999 for an inpatient palliative care unit through charitable activities like special events. The hospital raised another $2 million for Dr. Foley's chair. The consistent pursuit of clinical and research excellence has been critical in maintaining credibility and continued support for the Pain and Palliative Care Service in an environment where high-quality research and academic accomplishment are prized.

The Pain and Palliative Care Service has thrived, as well, because of support from many people in various services and departments. Collegial relationships and a shared dedication to improving patient care have permitted the Service to develop.

The Pain and Palliative Care Service at MSKCC is unique because of its relatively long and successful history. Many issues must be considered in establishing such programs and in providing a structure and foundation to make excellence possible. Here are a few of the most important factors.

Institutional Home for Pain and Palliative Care Programs

MSKCC is the only institution that now has a separate department for pain and palliative care. Without a separate department, an institution's leaders must establish policies and procedures, and create an environment, to support the faculty members leading the pain and palliative care program. To be truly interdisciplinary, the programs must be horizontally organized, and institutional leaders must have a thoughtful plan on how to administer the programs across traditional departmental lines. Otherwise the results are duplicated programs, lost opportunities for collaborative research, institutional confusion, and wasted money.

A palliative care program should be located wherever a given institution's strengths and resources lie. At MSKCC, this continues to be within the Department of Neurology. In other institutions, the appropriate home for a palliative care program may be within general internal medicine, oncology, geriatrics, or family medicine. Given the scope of skills and resources required to meet the clinical, spiritual, and emotional needs of patients and families, it is unlikely that a program can be housed primarily outside of the medical departments, in services such as anesthesiology or psychiatry, even though these two disciplines play key roles in pain management and palliative care.

When the pain and palliative care program is housed in a specific clinical department, administrative and academic mechanisms must provide joint appointments across departmental lines. To be effective, the program's leader(s) must be able to participate in evaluating faculty members and allocating resources.

Reimbursement and Faculty Compensation
Inadequate reimbursement constitutes a barrier to improved palliative care (Committee on Care..., 1997). Inadequate reimbursement for professional services is exacerbated in a true interdisciplinary environment, because only one physician may bill for a particular diagnosis. When the palliative care team urges highly paid, technically oriented physicians like anesthesiologists to limit procedures that the patient and family do not want, reimbursement tensions within an interdisciplinary service get worse. Moreover, it is unclear what criteria

should be used to determine physicians' compensation for palliative care, particularly for vital services that are traditionally reimbursed at relatively low rates.

Creating a freestanding hospital department of palliative medicine does not eliminate the problems of reimbursement and faculty compensation. Freestanding departments do have obvious potential benefits in providing unified, coherent clinical service and common standards of practice within the service, and they have a single leader who serves as a role model for palliative care within the institution. However, autonomous departments may paradoxically make it harder to recruit physicians who are unwilling or financially unable to leave their primary specialties, particularly without a specialty in palliative medicine or pain management approved by the American Board of Medical Specialties (ABMS). These reimbursement pressures can be moderated if an institution subsidizes palliative care services through clinical departments that generate higher revenues.

Finally, for pain management and palliative care services to survive and thrive in academic institutions, they must establish and maintain the same high standards of patient care, teaching, and research that all other services in an institution must meet. Otherwise, the other services will invariably see them as second-class operations.

I. Institutional Information

    A. Name of program: Pain and Palliative Care Service

    B. Program director: Richard Payne, MD, Chief of Service

    C. Date that the program began: 1981

    D. Institutional setting: Urban, acute care hospital

    E. Type of institution: NCI-designated comprehensive cancer center

    F. Number of beds: 454

    G. Health care system

        1. Number of hospital affiliates in the health care system: 0

        2. Number of long-term care affiliates in the health care system:

II. Program Characteristics

    A. Clinical Staff

        1. Physicians

            Richard Payne, Chief; Member and Attending Neurologist

            Kathleen Foley, Member and Attending Neurologist

            Gavril Pasternak, Member and Attending Neurologist (Neuroscientist)

            Gilbert Gonzales, Associate Attending Neurologist

            Eugenia Obbens, Associate Attending Neurologist

            Paulo Manfredi, Assistant Attending Neurologist

            Ricardo Cruciani, Assistant Attending Neuropharmacologist

            Alan Carver, Clinical Assistant Neurologist

        2. Nurses

            Nessa Coyle, ANP

            Mary Layman Goldstein, ANP

            Susan Derby, ANP

            Didi Loseth, CNS

            Bernadette Clark, RN

            Clara Grande-Cameron, ANP

        3. Social Workers

            Barbara Pollack

        4. Other health care providers

            Sherry Schacter, RN, PhD, Attending Bereavement and Grief Therapist

B. Research Staff

    1. Dedicated research staff: Yes

    2. Who they are:

        Ricardo Cruciani, MD, PhD, Assistant Neuropharmacologist

        Ann Radovitch, Research Coordinator, Data Manager

        Sarah Kless, Data Manager

        Charles Inturrisi, PhD, Professor of Pharmacology, Cornell Medical College

C. Administrative Staff

Freya Wigler, Administrative Coordinator

Melissa Adamson, Chief Office Assistant

Bridget King, Physician Office Assistant (Dr. Foley)

Theresa Rivera, Outpatient Clinic and Fellows Secretary

Lawrence Tavernier, Physician Office Assistant (Drs. Manfredi and Obbens)

D. Clinical Characteristics

Patient population: patients with pain and other symptoms associated with cancer or cancer therapy. Patients are seen at all stages of disease, from initial diagnosis through death.

    1. Hospital department or division:

        The Service is based in the Neurology Department of a hospital.

    2. Consult service:

        The Pain and Palliative Inpatient Consult Service sees patients referred by the nursing or physician staff 24 hours a day, 7 days a week.

    3. Dedicated inpatient palliative care unit: We have a 6-bed inpatient unit.

    4. Dedicated inpatient hospice unit: No. Patients are referred to local hospices.

    5. Home hospice program: No. The Supportive Care Program serves patients with difficult pain and symptom management problems who want to stay at home.

    6. Palliative care home-care program: No. The Supportive Care Program serves both patients who are being treated for their disease and those who are no longer receiving therapy.

E. Patient Population

    1. Number of patients per month in the inpatient unit: Our inpatient unit has been open only since February 1, 2000.

    2. Number of patients per month on consult service: Between 200 and

250 new inpatients.

3. Number of patients per month receiving home care: 12-15 patients are followed by each nurse in the Supportive Care Program at any given time.

4. Number of patients per month in hospice: N/A

5. Average length of stay in the program:

    a. Inpatient: Too new to determine.

    b. Outpatient: Ranges from 1 day to 15 years.

F. Estimated Funding Sources

    1. Foundation grants: 25%

    2. Federal grants: 5%

    3. Endowments: 5%

    4. Charity: 0

    5. Hospital support: 65%

    6. Medical school support: 0

    7. Clinical income: 0

    8. Other sources: 0

G. Educational Component

    1. Program types

        a. Administrative coordinator: 1 (institutional support)

        b. Medical secretaries: 4 (institutional support)

        c. Clinic secretary: 1 (institutional support)

    2. Trainees

        a. Fellows: 5 (philanthropic support)

        b. Residents: 0

        c. Medical students: third-year students at Weill Medical College do a two-week rotation on the Service. Approximately 4 medical students from other institutions do one-month rotations on the Service.

        d. Faculty: 5 (supported by institutional/practice funds)

        e. Nurses: 2 advanced practice nurses conduct consultations and educational sessions throughout the hospital (institutional support)

        1 nurse practitioner in the inpatient unit (philanthropic support)

        3 advanced practice nurses in Supportive Care Program. One of the nurses is a certified grief therapist and conducts group and individual sessions with

patients and families.

1 research nurse (philanthropic and industrial support)

f. Social worker: 1 (institutional support)

g. Public: 0

h. Observers: approximately 25-30 per year. Some of these visitors come through the Network Project supported by NCI funds. Others are invited by the Service.

III. Research Component: Funding sources

A. Federal grants: 10%

B. Foundation grants: 40%

C. Industry: 50%

D. Intramural: 0%

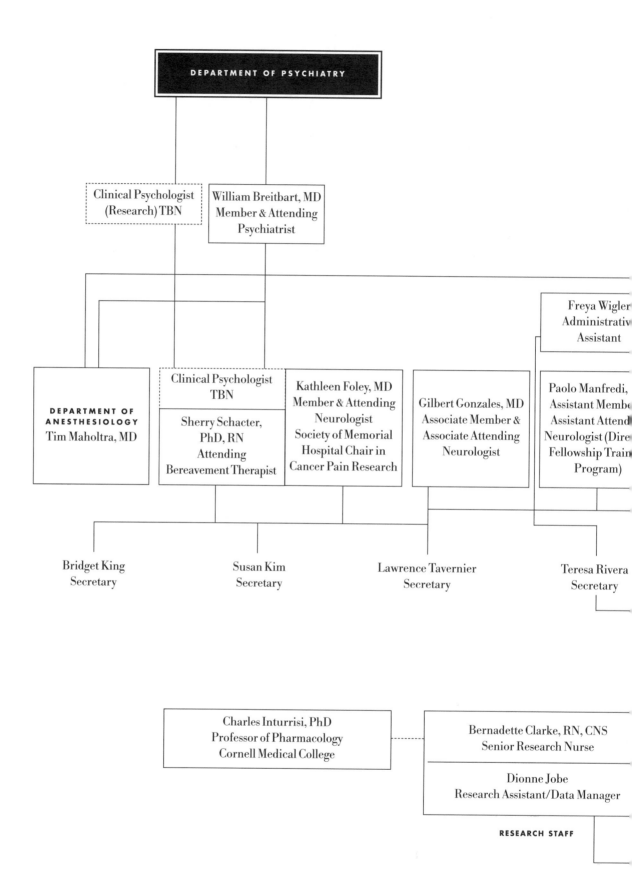

DEPARTMENT OF PSYCHIATRY

Clinical Psychologist (Research) TBN

William Breitbart, MD
Member & Attending Psychiatrist

Freya Wigler
Administrative Assistant

DEPARTMENT OF ANESTHESIOLOGY
Tim Maholtra, MD

Clinical Psychologist TBN

Sherry Schacter, PhD, RN
Attending Bereavement Therapist

Kathleen Foley, MD
Member & Attending Neurologist
Society of Memorial Hospital Chair in Cancer Pain Research

Gilbert Gonzales, MD
Associate Member & Associate Attending Neurologist

Paolo Manfredi,
Assistant Member
Assistant Attending
Neurologist (Director
Fellowship Training
Program)

Bridget King
Secretary

Susan Kim
Secretary

Lawrence Tavernier
Secretary

Teresa Rivera
Secretary

Charles Inturrisi, PhD
Professor of Pharmacology
Cornell Medical College

Bernadette Clarke, RN, CNS
Senior Research Nurse

Dionne Jobe
Research Assistant/Data Manager

RESEARCH STAFF

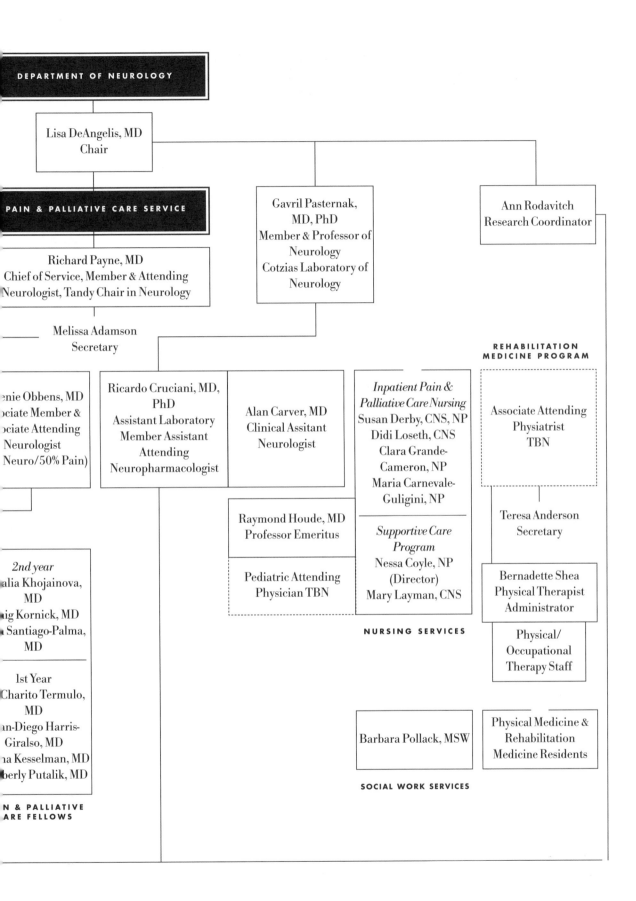

Lisa DeAngelis, MD
Chair

PAIN & PALLIATIVE CARE SERVICE

Richard Payne, MD
Chief of Service, Member & Attending
Neurologist, Tandy Chair in Neurology

Gavril Pasternak,
MD, PhD
Member & Professor of
Neurology
Cotzias Laboratory of
Neurology

Ann Rodavitch
Research Coordinator

Melissa Adamson
Secretary

REHABILITATION
MEDICINE PROGRAM

enie Obbens, MD
ociate Member &
ociate Attending
Neurologist
Neuro/50% Pain)

Ricardo Cruciani, MD,
PhD
Assistant Laboratory
Member Assistant
Attending
Neuropharmacologist

Alan Carver, MD
Clinical Assitant
Neurologist

Inpatient Pain &
Palliative Care Nursing
Susan Derby, CNS, NP
Didi Loseth, CNS
Clara Grande-
Cameron, NP
Maria Carnevale-
Guligini, NP

Associate Attending
Physiatrist
TBN

Raymond Houde, MD
Professor Emeritus

Teresa Anderson
Secretary

Supportive Care
Program
Nessa Coyle, NP
(Director)
Mary Layman, CNS

Pediatric Attending
Physician TBN

Bernadette Shea
Physical Therapist
Administrator

2nd year
alia Khojainova,
MD
ig Kornick, MD
Santiago-Palma,
MD

Physical/
Occupational
Therapy Staff

NURSING SERVICES

1st Year
Charito Termulo,
MD
an-Diego Harris-
Giralso, MD
na Kesselman, MD
erly Putalik, MD

Barbara Pollack, MSW

Physical Medicine &
Rehabilitation
Medicine Residents

N & PALLIATIVE
ARE FELLOWS

SOCIAL WORK SERVICES

RACE

Asian Indian	2%
Asian	1%
Black Hispanic	1%
Black Non-Hispanic	11%
White Hispanic	7%
White Non-Hispanic	75%
Unknown/Other	2%

GENDER

Female	58%
Male	42%

LOCALE

Local (NY, NJ, CT)	90%
Nonlocal USA	6%
International	3%

CAUSE OF PAIN

Cancer	80%
Treatment	14%
Unrelated	4%
No pain	2%

TYPE OF PAIN

Bony	38%
Soft Tissue	26%
Visceral	16%
Nerve	5%
Other	4%
Unreported	11%

SITE OF PAIN

Abdomen	30%
Head and Neck	17%
Back	16%
Pelvis/Perineum	16%
Leg	8%
Arm	4%
Chest Wall	4%
Hip	1%
Other	3%
Unreported	1%

CANCER

Lung	12.0%
Breast	7.5%
Colorectal	7.5%
Sarcoma	7.5%
Lymphoma, non-Hodgkin's	4.5%
Pancreas	4.5%
Prostate	4.5%
Acute myelocytic leukemia	3.0%
Head and neck	3.0%
Melanoma	3.0%
Ovary	3.0%
Stomach	3.0%
Uterus	3.0%
Cervical	2.0%
Acute lymphocytic leukemia	1.5%
Chronic myelocytic leukemia	1.5%
Connective tissue	1.5%
Endometrium	1.5%
Gallbladder	1.5%
Nasopharynx	1.5%
Neuroblastoma	1.5%
Other	21.5%

PHARMACOLOGIC INTERVENTIONS

Opioid start	5%
Opioid increase	21%
Opioid decrease	4%
Opioid rotation	33%
No change	10%
Unknown	27%

OTHER INTERVENTIONS

Palliative physician	46%
Nursing	24%
Referral-psychiatry	13%
Social work	8%
Discharge	2%
Prognosis/goals of care	2%
Referral–Anesthesia Pain Service	2%
Referral–Neurology	1%
Withhold or withdraw treatment	1%
DNR	1%
Clergy	0%
Grief specialist	0%
Health care proxy	0%
Living will	0%
Sedation	0%

Memorial Sloan-Kettering Cancer Center

Funding Sources*

Hospital Support	65%	■
Foundation Grants	25%	▧
Endowments	5%	◩
Federal Grants**	5%	◼

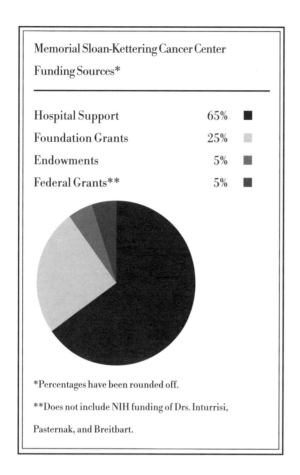

*Percentages have been rounded off.

**Does not include NIH funding of Drs. Inturrisi,

Pasternak, and Breitbart.

RESEARCH PROJECTS

Topical Levorphanol and Lidocaine for Pain Associated with Chemotherapy-induced Mucositis
Primary investigator (PI): Paolo Manfredi, MD
Supported by EpiCent Pharmaceuticals

Celecoxib for Paclitaxel-induced Arthritis and Myalgias
PI: Gilbert Gonzales, MD
Sponsored by Searle

Valdecoxib in Chronic Cancer Pain
PI: Eugenie Obbens, MD
Sponsored by Searle

A Prospective Study of the Impact of Pain Management on the Prevalence of Depressed and
Anxious Mood and Will to Live in a Population of Patients with Cancer Pain
PIs: Sean O'Mahony, MD, and Richard Payne, MD

Rehabilitative Needs Assessment of Breast Cancer Patients
PIs: Andrea Cheville, MD, and Richard Payne, MD
Sponsored by Langeloth Foundation

Quality of Life and Outcomes of Patients Treated in Palliative Care Programs in the Tri-State
Area: A Pilot Study of the Palliative Care Outcomes Consortium
PI: Richard Payne, MD
Memorial Sloan Kettering Cancer Center

Retrospective Central Pain Study
PI: Gilbert Gonzales, MD
Memorial Sloan-Kettering Cancer Center

Development of a Pain and Palliative Care Program at North General Hospital

PI: Richard Payne, MD

Supported by NGH, MSKCC, Robert Wood Johnson Foundation, and Ellen P. Hermanson
Foundation

Educate staff regarding pain management and palliative care, organize a program to meet
patients' needs, and hire an advanced practice nurse to anchor new program.

Harlem Palliative Care Network

PI: Richard Payne, MD

Supported by United Hospital Fund. The Fan Fox and Leslie R. Samuels Foundation and the
U.S. Department of Commerce are being approached for additional support.

MSKCC, the Visiting Nurse Service, and North General Hospital direct this palliative care
project to improve the quality of life for Harlem residents facing life-threatening illnesses.

Catholic Health Care System Community Palliative Care Network

PI: Richard Payne, MD

Supported by a grant from the United Hospital Fund. Participants include Calvary Hospital,
Catholic Charities, Vividus Cancer Care Network, New York Medical College, and MSKCC.
This organization of hospitals, nursing homes and affiliated health care institutions was
formed to coordinate the delivery of palliative care to patients in New York City and in
Westchester, Dutchess, Ulster, Orange, Rockland, and Putnam counties.

Initiative to Improve Palliative and End of Life Care in the African-American Community

PIs: Richard Payne, MD, and Harold Freeman, MD

Supported by Project on Death in America, Robert Wood Johnson Foundation, the Milbank
Memorial Fund, North General Hospital, and MSKCC.

A selected group of African-American professionals will meet in a series of sessions to identify
the historic, religious, and sociocultural factors that have affected many African Americans'
use of palliative care and pain management.

Psychiatric and Pain Research Training in Cancer
PI: Richard Payne, MD, and Jamie Ostroff, PhD
Sponsored by NIH
A federal training grant that supports research by psychiatry and pain fellows.

Biochemical Characterization of Opioid Binding Sites
PI: Gavril Pasternak, MD, PhD
Sponsored by NIH

Pharmacology and Neuroscience of Drug Abuse
PIs: Charles Inturrisi, PhD, and Richard Payne, MD
Sponsored by NIDA/NIH

REFERENCES

Breitbart, W., M. McDonald, B. Rosenfeld, N.D. Monkman, and S. Passik. 1998. Fatigue in Ambulatory AIDS Patients. *Journal of Pain and Symptom Management*, 15(159):167.

Committee on Care at the End of Life of the Institute of Medicine. 1997. *Approaching Death: Improving Care at the End of Life*, eds. M. Field and C. Cassel. Washington, D.C.: National Academy Press.

Coyle, N. 1989. Continuity of Care for the Cancer Patient with Chronic Pain. *Cancer*, 63:2289–93.

Coyle, N. 1995. Supportive Care Program, Pain Service, Memorial Sloan-Kettering Cancer Center. *Supportive Care in Cancer*, 3:161–3.

Fishman, B., et al. 1987. The Memorial Pain Assessment Card: A Valid Instrument for the Evaluation of Cancer Pain. *Cancer*, 60:1151–8.

Foley, K.M. 1979. Pain Syndromes in Patients with Cancer. *Advances in Pain Research and Therapy*, 2:59–75.

Foley, K.M., C.E. Inturrisi. 1986. *Advances in Pain Research and Therapy: Opioid Analgesics in the Management of Clinical Pain*. New York: Raven Press.

Foley, K.M., C.E. Inturrisi, I. Kourides, R.F. Kaiko, J. Posner, R. Houde, et al. 1978. Intravenous (IV) and Intraventricular (IVT) Administration of Beta Endorphin (Bzh-EP) in Man: Safety and Disposition. In *Characteristics and Function of Opioids*, eds. J. Van Ree and L. Terenius, 421–2. Amsterdam: Elsevier/North Holland Biomedical Press.

Foley, K.M., V. Ventafridda, and J.J. Bonica. 1990. *Proceedings of the Second International Congress on Cancer Pain*. New York: Raven Press.

Houde, R.W., S.L. Wallenstein, and A. Rogers. 1960. Clinical Pharmacology of Analgesics: 1. A Method for Studying Analgesic Effect. *Clinical Pharmacology and Therapeutics*, 1:163–74.

Kaiko, R.F., K.M. Foley, R. Houde, and C.E. Inturrisi. 1978. Narcotic Levels in Cerebrospinal Fluid and Plasma in Man. In *Characteristics and Function of Opioids*, eds. J. Van Ree and L. Terenius, 221–2. Amsterdam: Elsevier/North-Holland Biomedical Press.

Kuhar, M., and G.W. Pasternak. 1983. *Analgesics: Neurochemical, Behavioral, and Chemical Properties*. New York: Raven Press.

Payne, R., J. Madson, R. Harvey, and C. Inturrisi. 1986. A Chronic Sheep Preparation for the Study of Pharmacokinetics of Opiate Drugs. *Journal of Pharmacological Methods*, 16:277–96.

Payne, R., R.B. Patt, and C.S. Hill. 1998. *Assessment and Treatment of Cancer Pain*. Seattle: International Association of the Study of Pain Press.

Portenoy, R.K., H.T. Thaler, A.B. Kornblith, et al. 1994. The Memorial Symptom Assessment Scale: An Instrument for Evaluation of Symptom Prevalence, Characteristics and Distress. *European Journal of Cancer*, 30A(9):1326–36.

Rosenfeld, B, W. Breitbart, K. Stein, J. Funesti-Esch, M. Kaim, and S.G.M. Krivo. 1999. Measuring Desire for Death among Patients with HIV/AIDS: The Schedule of Attitudes toward Hastened Death. *American Journal of Psychiatry*, 156:94–100.

Strassels, S., D. Carr, M. Meldrum, and M.J. Cousins. 1999. Toward a Canon of the Pain and Analgesia Literature: A Citation Analysis. *Current Researches in Anesthesia and Analgesia*, 89:1528–33.

World Health Organization (WHO). 1986. *Cancer Pain Relief*. Geneva.

WHO Expert Committee. 1990. *Cancer Pain Relief and Palliative Care*. WHO Technical Reports Series, no. 804. Geneva.

WHO. 1998. *Cancer Pain Relief and Palliative Care in Children*. Geneva: World Health Organization (in collaboration with The International Association of the Study of Pain).

The Lilian and Benjamin Hertzberg Palliative Care Institute, Mount Sinai School of Medicine

Diane E. Meier, Jane Morris, and R. Sean Morrison

Why We Do This Work

People often ask those of us in the Palliative Care Program at Mount Sinai how we can bear to do such difficult, emotionally demanding work. So much loss. So much suffering and death. In response, one of us recently pointed out that loss, anguish, and death were all around us long before we began palliative care. Back then, our own suffering as professionals grew out of our distress at how little was being done about the physical, emotional, and existential problems of our patients and their families. We saw firsthand how well-intentioned but wrong-headed much of the care seemed to be. We shared an escalating sense of frustration but felt helpless to alter the situation. Finally, our experience with one patient whose story was published in the *New England Journal of Medicine** helped transform distress and frustration into action. This 73-year-old man with terminal cancer spent 47 days in an acute care hospital, where he eventually died. In the hospital, he endured investigative tests and was tied to his bed for 29 days, despite his and his family's desire to reject further diagnostic intervention and life-prolonging treatment. We knew that this man and others like him suffer needlessly at the end of life. Developing the Palliative Care Program has reduced our own professional suffering by giving us tools and opportunities to improve care for our patients and by allowing us to show colleagues and students another way of caring for patients with serious or life-threatening illness.

How We Got Started

The Catalysts

Four core faculty members began the Palliative Care Program at the Mount Sinai School of Medicine in 1997: Drs. Diane E. Meier, R. Sean Morrison, and Judith C. Ahronheim, and Jane Morris, M.S., R.N. The following factors were critical to the program's development and successes:

1. External, primarily foundation-based, funding for faculty development and clinical program development—as opposed to empirical research funding—permitted the core faculty to devote the required time to the project and established palliative medicine as a legitimate academic pursuit.

2. Colleagues in the Department of Geriatrics, three doctors and a nurse, conceptualized and launched the

---

* R.S. Morrison, D.E. Meier, and C.K. Cassel. "When Too Much is Too Little," *New England Journal of Medicine* 335 (1996):1755–9.

program. They shared a commitment to the program, worked well together, and were able to distribute the responsibilities of the new program so that no one person was shouldering the entire load.

3. Our program enjoys highly supportive and powerful institutional leadership and mentoring, primarily from our department chair but also from the dean of the Medical School and the president/CEO of the Hospital and Health System. Their efforts facilitated repeated exposure to the broader community and helped us reach segments of the Mount Sinai community that were traditionally resistant, like oncology.

4. In an academic medical center, the status of the principal palliative care faculty as respected clinicians, teachers, and researchers contributed to our acceptance and integration into the medical school and hospital.

5. Through patient–doctor contacts and subsequent development of relationships, several benefactors have donated generously to the palliative care program. Donors have committed a substantial endowment for a Palliative Care Institute. An endowment for an annual lecture in palliative care has brought national leaders in the field to Mount Sinai, bringing institutional and citywide publicity for our work. Many smaller donors have also contributed to the program. This support has permitted vital travel and education for our clinical faculty, allowed the hiring of research staff, and supplied financial reserves for the growth of the program.

Barriers

The major threats to the program's survival are financial. The fiscal environment in New York City teaching hospitals makes it nearly impossible to obtain hospital operations budget support for the program's clinical services. Billing income covers approximately 10 percent of clinical costs. The rest of the staff's salaries and benefits come from overlapping foundation and federal grants and from philanthropy. The head of nursing at our hospital recently agreed to cover 50 percent of the nurse coordinator's position and is considering covering 50 percent of a second nurse to be hired soon. Salaries for physicians, researchers, and support staff are paid primarily from grants. We do not have enough money to hire a social worker, volunteer-program coordinator, or pastoral counselor. The risks of continued undercapitalization include understaffing, burnout, and inability to provide high-quality clinical and educational services. We have concentrated on obtaining endowment funding in an effort to secure the program's long-term existence.

 Inspiration and Motivation

Rising frustration among the core faculty at the gap between what patients needed and what they actually received from doctors and nurses inspired the program. Experiences with patients like the one described in the *New England Journal of Medicine* and with patients who had advanced Alzheimer's disease showed the urgent need to change the patterns of care and the education of medical professionals. The support for faculty development from the Faculty Scholars Program of the Project on Death in America was critical in letting us translate motivation into action. This program, which identifies and supports academic leaders in palliative medicine at teaching hospitals, provided not only salaries but also a network of professional colleagues engaged in the same work, facing similar challenges, elsewhere. Leaders of the Faculty Scholars Program also provided consistent, concrete mentoring during the development of our program, on issues like negotiation strategies, teaching skills, and the emotional impact of working in this field. The Faculty Scholars Program was a key to our confidence in what we were undertaking and to our successes.

Through our Faculty Scholars award, the four people who began our program developed a seminar series in palliative care for other faculty members—a teach-the-teachers model of continuing education. We believed that effective training of students and residents began with the examples set by their teachers and mentors. Since our colleagues had not been trained in palliative medicine, we started a series of twice-monthly seminars focused on the needs of clinical faculty. This faculty development curriculum ranged from the basic pharmacology of pain management to physician countertransference issues in caring for the dying. We recruited participants to the seminars based on both objective and subjective criteria. We invited faculty from the specialties most involved with seriously ill patients—oncology, neurology, pulmonary care, critical care, pediatric oncology, geriatrics, and general medicine. We sought out the highly respected teachers, clinicians, and opinion leaders in those specialties. We hoped for a positive response from 10 or 20 faculty members and were surprised and gratified when almost all the people we contacted said that they wanted to participate.

Many colleagues expressed relief that we were trying to provide tools they needed when addressing the symptoms and communication needs of their sickest patients. Approximately 60 full-time faculty ultimately participated in the seminar along with 20 to 30 colleagues in nursing, social work, legal affairs, risk management, and ethics. Thus, the PDIA-funded faculty development seminar series let us introduce the principles of palliative medicine near the end of life to colleagues from diverse specialties within the medical center. In addition, we developed a collegial network within the hospital and medical school, connections that have furthered the growth of our program. Some participants in the seminars have become close colleagues as consultants on individual cases, as research collaborators, and as clinical faculty in the palliative care program. Starting with professional development and team building before initiating any clinical service has turned out to be essential to the acceptance and growth of our clinical and teaching service.

 Acceptance by Colleagues
. . . .

Referrals from new attending physicians and new clinical departments continue to increase. For example, the last few months of 1999 have seen a dramatic rise in referrals by the neurosurgical ICU of patients in coma or persistent vegetative state. But several barriers persist. Many colleagues still see palliative care as brink-of-death care and fail to appreciate its value earlier in the course of a serious illness. Therefore, we are often

consulted on patients only days or weeks before death, long after important opportunities to manage symptoms, communicate with family members, and complete important tasks have passed. In response to this persistent phenomenon, we are trying simultaneously to teach life prolonging *and* palliative care to our house staff, students, and attending physicians.

Second, the oncology service at Mount Sinai was initially unreceptive to our program and saw no role for palliative care for their patients and families. The new division chief of oncology, however, is an advocate of palliative medicine, and she strongly supports a collaboration with our group. In a recent encouraging development, the oncology division has begun requiring all hematology-oncology fellows to rotate on the palliative care service. We are optimistic that her leadership will eventually effect the change that we could not accomplish alone.

Program Development
. . . .

Initial Goals
The purpose of the program is educational. The clinical service exists to teach medical and nursing professionals, at their patients' bedsides, to deliver the highest quality of care in the face of a serious illness and near the end of life. Because Mount Sinai is a

teaching hospital, students and house staff from diverse specialties care for virtually all patients on the consultation and inpatient services. We are convinced that this is the most effective, lasting kind of education, one that shapes the knowledge and attitudes of doctors in training far more than any lecture. We also deliver lectures and case-based sessions to the house staff and nursing staff in both home care and inpatient settings, and to attending physicians.

Key Steps in Program Development at Mount Sinai

We identified a group of interested faculty members, created a core team, and distributed responsibilities among these individuals. Team members prepared themselves through training at Memorial Sloan-Kettering and elsewhere, visits to established clinical–academic programs at Northwestern University and Cleveland Clinic, and intensive self-education.

To persuade colleagues that improved palliative care was needed, we held faculty and staff training seminars for 18 months before clinical services began. We conducted a study to assess the pain of hospitalized patients. We presented the data, which revealed widespread undertreatment on several units, to targeted audiences. We delivered grand rounds in all major clinical departments of the medical center.

We met regularly with major hospital and medical school administrators and leaders to provide updated information, to seek advice, and to build support in the constituency most likely to influence the program's future. We prepared the medical center to expect our new service through extensive hospital and community publicity. The Service was introduced by letters from the president and CEO of the hospital, letters from the head of nursing and social work, and direct mailings to every physician, house officer, medical student, nurse, social worker, hospital administrator, and trustee associated with the medical center.

We applied successfully for foundation funding for salaries, faculty development, and program start-up costs and have continued applying for research funding in diverse areas of palliative medicine. We have sought publications in professional journals and have taken part in national meetings and leadership functions.

Our successful consultations have led to more consultations. After its first two years, the palliative care service is considered almost as routine as many other sources of consultation in the hospital. We hired a full-time neurologist, who had trained in a pain fellowship, to ensure expert consultation. This not only provided excellent patient care but also convinced our colleagues that we offered something that they themselves could not provide.

We have developed a patient database. For palliative programs like Mount Sinai's to set the standard of care, the medical community must have detailed information about their nature and content. Our database quantifies patient information, symptom burden, recommended intervention, implementation or lack of it, reasons for lack of implementation, and outcomes of the intervention. The interventions catalogued include recommendations for analgesics, family meetings, and decisions about withholding or withdrawing life-sustaining treatments. Keeping the database current requires daily participation by the nurse and doctor on the clinical consultation team as well as a research assistant and data manager–programmer. Database development has helped us to explain exactly what we mean by palliative care, report on what we do, and identify areas that need improvement.

We have created support for the program throughout the hospital by educating the hospital community about the many ways that a strong palliative care program benefits the institution. The obvious fiscal argument, that palliative care saves money by reducing length of stay and ancillary expenses, has been an effective approach at some other institutions and has recently begun to get a hearing at Mount Sinai. Palliative care can help the hospital

financially. Most people agree that palliative care is compassionate for dying patients and their families and that identifying such patients and either helping them to go home, as most patients prefer, or to go to other appropriate settings like long-term care or hospice will lead to substantial savings. Analyzing all adult deaths for a fiscal year for length of stay, costs and charges, and actual reimbursement is an instructive exercise for hospital administrators. The mean and median length of stay for patients who ultimately die in the hospital is two to three times longer than the average length of stay, and reimbursement for these patients falls far short of costs.

Even though the fiscal argument can be convincing, it can be risky to advocate palliative care primarily on that basis. Patients, family members, and the public may interpret such advocacy as evidence that palliative care means letting people die rather than trying to prolong their lives, or trying to discharge them from the hospital instead of continuing to provide expensive inpatient care. Second, it is difficult to demonstrate that the savings actually occur. It is neither ethically nor practically possible to randomize patients in order to compare palliative and traditional care. Furthermore, patients referred to the palliative care service are not comparable to other seriously ill inpatients. Palliative care referrals tend to involve the sickest patients who stay longest, and clarity about the goals of their care is often elusive. There may be other fiscal savings. Ancillary spending may be reduced if the length of stay remains long but fewer procedures and tests are ordered. Referrals of inpatients to certified home health agencies, hospices, and other physicians may increase. In our view, however, the fiscal argument should be secondary to the quality of care as a justification for hospital-based palliative care programs. Palliative care for patients and families facing serious and distressing illness should become the standard of practice. We cannot claim to be providing good care to our sickest patients unless we are also providing palliative care.

Program development should include the appropriate structure. A hospital-based palliative care program can begin with a consultative model, a dedicated inpatient unit, or both. Mount Sinai began with a hospital-wide consultation service. We wanted to send the message that palliative care is the responsibility of every doctor and nurse on every service, and not something to be relegated to a specialist or to a physically separate and potentially marginal unit. We thought we would have the widest educational impact by caring for patients as consultants, working *with* primary attendings, house staff, and nurses throughout the hospital, rather than

supplanting them. This model suited our educational goals.

In 1998 we decided to add a four-bed inpatient unit. These beds are part of a general medicine teaching ward, so that all palliative care inpatients are cared for by medicine house staff and students, who receive an intensive exposure to palliative care patients and skills. The unit has been useful in extending our consultation base to the ICUs and emergency department, since the unit is seen as an appropriate place for many patients in those areas. We are considering raising funds for an expanded and remodeled unit with amenities such as furniture, lamps, single rooms, and privacy. Such a unit would increase the visibility and credibility of our service within the larger medical center and would symbolize the importance and permanence of palliative care.

One disadvantage of establishing a physically distinct inpatient unit, however, is that clinicians may come to view palliative care as an isolated specialty rather than as a body of knowledge and skills that every clinician should have and use. Inpatient units also create their own inverse incentives and momentum. Once the beds are established, you have to keep them filled or risk losing them. The pressure to keep beds filled may not always lead to decisions based solely on patients' best interests. Yet combined hospice, palliative care inpatient programs, and consultation services, like those at Northwestern University, have enjoyed substantial financial stability because inpatient and hospice revenues essentially pay the personnel costs of the consult service.

Program development requires an interdisciplinary clinical team. The Mount Sinai clinical palliative care team currently consists of two full-time nurse specialists with master's degrees; a rotating series of attending physicians that equal one FTE, and research and administrative staff. Geriatrics and oncology fellows are assigned to the service for one-month mandatory rotations. Residents and medical students rotate on an elective basis. Staff social workers assigned to individual inpatient units provide social work services. In addition, the Department of Social Work has designated a senior social work faculty member as liaison to the Palliative Care Program. The hospital chaplaincy program is called upon case by case.

Effective physician staffing is essential. Mount Sinai chose a multispecialty attending physician model. Attending physicians rotate on the palliative care consultation service for one month each year. At present, there are 12 attending physicians, half of whom are geriatricians. The rest are from oncology, general medicine, the AIDS service, and pulmonary–critical care. None of us, including the physicians who lead the program, were trained in palliative care fellowships. We learned the basics of palliative medicine by intensive independent study, greatly stimulated by having to teach others; by brief rotations at established pain and palliative care programs, including Memorial Sloan-Kettering's Network Observer Project, Northwestern University, and Cleveland Clinic; training through the AMA's program on Educating Physicians in End of Life Care (EPEC); and by taking care of patients.

When we encounter difficult pain problems, we call upon consultants from the pain service for neurolytic blocks, epidural infusions, and other procedures for refractory symptoms. This model has worked well, at least in part because the vast majority of what we do is palliative care, meaning care of seriously ill and dying patients, and not chronic pain management such as chronic headache, low-back pain, and work-related injuries. In addition, the most time-consuming and challenging clinical issues common to palliative care have to do with establishing the goals of medical care and ensuring good communication among the principals on a plan of care for the patient. In general, physical symptoms and their treatment tend to be the clearest, most straightforward part of the patient's management.

In practice, a new attending physician begins the rotation by working with a more experienced colleague, goes to as many training sessions as possible, like the EPEC program, and relies a great deal upon the sophisticated knowledge and experience of our clinical director, Jane Morris. What we give up in depth of expertise and credentials, we gain in the rapid growth of a cadre of medical school faculty with knowledge, experience, and teaching and research interests in palliative medicine. These attendings become the experts in palliative medicine within their own divisions and departments, and continue to teach and model palliative care precepts wherever they work, not merely during their palliative service rotation. As the field develops further and issues such as specialty status and board certification become more pressing, we may have to rethink this model. For the moment, this wide distribution of clinical and teaching responsibilities among attending physicians has enabled rapid growth of the program, minimized physicians' burnout, and created a rich multispecialty intellectual environment that fosters collaborative research and teaching throughout the medical center. In the future, our legitimacy as a service and a discipline will require a faculty member with pain fellowship training, who is interested in working with palliative care patients as opposed to chronic pain or postoperative pain patients.

We need to establish continuity of care. In a tertiary care teaching hospital, fragmentation, multiple specialists, and discontinuity characterize medical care. The seriously ill patient admitted to the hospital may or may not have a primary care doctor. Typically, the patient leaves the hospital with an appointment at an office that is all but impossible to visit under the burden imposed by the illness, may receive short-term nursing visits for a few weeks after discharge, and is then left alone to sink or swim through telephone contact with one or more busy specialists. It is no exaggeration to say that the health care system abandons many seriously ill patients when they go home. Approximately 17 percent of all adults are referred to hospice before death; in that case, they typically switch to an entirely new team of nurses and doctors for the last weeks or months of life. A hospital-based palliative care team cannot hope to reverse all of these entrenched discontinuities, but it should create a safety net for palliative care patients discharged from the hospital. Mount Sinai makes extensive efforts to establish a safe long-term plan of care in the community for every palliative care patient who survives to leave the hospital, through referrals to certified home-health agencies, hospice, or long-term care settings.

When Mount Sinai's palliative care patients are discharged, we give them the palliative care service beeper number so that they can reach the attending physician or nurse coordinator on call 24 hours a day, seven days a week. This continuity and contact does not replace the primary care doctor. But it serves as supplemental support to patient and family, often on symptom management, supervision of home care or hospice nurses, and provision of essential aid to families during periods of clinical instability and high stress. The Palliative Care Program has established a close working relationship with the Mount Sinai Certified Home Health Agency, which provides home care services for palliative care patients ineligible for, or unwilling to, transfer to hospice. This kind of round the clock coverage requires sufficient staff, another advantage of our multispecialty model for attending physicians.

These factors were the most helpful to us as we planned Mount Sinai's palliative care program:

- adequate funding
- a critical mass of people to share the work
- a high-quality product
- at least a minimal database
- allies in hospital administration, nursing, and medical records
- fund-raising skills

- staff time protected from other administrative and clinical responsibilities to let the program's leaders devote themselves to developing it, especially in the start-up phase

The following elements, which we did not have, would have helped us start the program:

- a business plan
- a proposal resource bank with transposable boilerplate language about palliative care and alternative program structures to choose from
- a strong fiscal argument citing data from other palliative care programs at other institutions

Challenges to the Program

As noted earlier, the major challenge to the growth and success of the program is financial. Inadequate clinical reimbursement and lack of hospital operations financing for the clinical service components impose constraints. Other barriers include the following:

1. Fear and denial of death among health professionals, patients and families can lead to the rejection of palliative care that is clearly needed.

2. There are emotional and psychological costs to the clinical and teaching doctors and nurses who experience repeated cycles of attachment and loss

of patients and families. Burnout and turnover of experienced staff are a serious risk.

3. Finding and recruiting faculty trained in pain management and palliative medicine is a national problem rooted in the paucity of training programs in this new specialty. The consequences include understaffing, exhaustion, and adverse impact on the quality of clinical and educational services.

4. Development of links with high-quality hospice programs in New York City continues to be a challenge. We are currently preparing a business plan with the hospital administration that would allow a direct contract with a local hospice for inpatient hospice beds. A contract would theoretically allow dying, hospitalized patients to be transferred from Medicare part A to the Medicare hospice benefit while still in the hospital, thereby serving the hospital's fiscal interests, and would facilitate safe and appropriate discharges to home hospice care, thereby serving the hospice's fiscal interests. Our home care agency has been unable to begin its own hospice program because we cannot obtain a certificate of need from New York State; there are already five hospices in the greater New York metropolitan area. An

in- and outpatient hospice relationship should enhance our teaching capabilities by exposing trainees to hospice, while increasing the timely, high-quality, compassionate care available to our patients and their families in the community.

5. Primary physicians are often legitimately concerned that palliative care consultation threatens their relationship to the patient. To assuage these concerns, we have taken extreme care to clear all our plans and recommendations with the primary physician before proposing them to the patient and family, and certainly before carrying them out. Ours is a consultative service, a model familiar to all physicians who practice in hospitals. The palliative care service assumes a primary care role only if the primary physician requests it.

6. Related turf issues involve institutional confusion about whom to call for pain problems in the hospital—the anesthesia pain service or the palliative care service. There are additional concerns about competition for the same patients and about threats to funding streams. We have found it important to be sensitive to these issues in order to prevent misunderstandings and antipathy toward the program.

Future Sustainability of the Program

Our current goal is to create a financial structure that will assure the existence of the program far into the future. The program cannot depend on grants, reimbursements, or hospital and medical school budgets, all of which are unstable sources of funding. Grants fund research projects, but clinical and educational activities have no routine, reliable sources of support. On the advice of the dean of our School of Medicine, we have embarked on a major search for philanthropic support for palliative care, intended to build an endowment large enough to cover the clinical and administrative costs of a clinical and teaching program. In the fall of 1999, our program was renamed the Lilian and Benjamin Hertzberg Palliative Care Institute to acknowledge a generous gift to the endowment fund. We are considering hiring a part-time development advisor to help raise money in a professional manner.

Institutional Culture

Key characteristics of our institutional culture that have facilitated the program's development include its academic orientation, the high profile of geriatric medicine in our medical center, and the national leadership roles and visibility of our department chair and medical center president. Institutional barriers include the highly specialized, fragmented nature of a tertiary care teaching hospital and its adverse effect on coherent delivery of, and teaching about, palliative medicine; the low priority accorded to clinical palliative care services compared to other clinical services in our hospital's budget, and the growing fiscal crisis afflicting our medical center during the last several years.

I. Institutional Information

    A. Name of Program: The Lilian and Benjamin Hertzberg Palliative Care Institute

    B. Program Director: Diane E. Meier, MD

    C. Program start-date: Palliative Care Seminar Series began in the fall of 1995. Consult service began July 1, 1997.

    D. Institutional setting: Urban

    E. Type of Institution: Academic

        1. Affiliated medical school: Mount Sinai School of Medicine

        2. Affiliated residency training program: Englewood Hospital, Elmhurst Hospital, Queens Hospital, Bronx VA Hospital, the Jewish Home and Hospital

    F. Number of beds: 1,110

    G. Health Care System

        1. Number of hospital affiliates in health care system: 25

        2. Number of long-term care affiliates in health care system: 13

II. Program Characteristics

    A. Clinical Staff

        1. Physicians' specialties

            Diane E. Meier (geriatrics/medicine, bioethics, palliative medicine)

            R. Sean Morrison (geriatrics/medicine, bioethics, palliative medicine)

            Roger Waltzman (oncology/medicine)

            John Carter (geriatrics/medicine)

            Cynthia Pan (geriatrics/medicine)

            Tobe Banc (geriatrics/medicine)

            Jeremy Boal (general medicine/geriatrics, home care, medical education)

            Stacie Pinderhughes (geriatrics/medicine)

            Sonni Mun (general medicine)

            David Muller (general medicine)

            Rainier Soriano (geriatrics/medicine)

            Judith Nelson (pulmonary/critical care)

            Valerie Parkas (HIV-AIDS/medicine)

        2. Nurses

            Jane Morris, MS, RN

Eileen Chichin, RN, DSW

    3.   Social Worker

        Felice Zilberfein, PhD

    4.   Other Health Care Providers (none)

B.   Research Staff

    Suzy Goldhirsch, MA: research coordinator

    Dana Natale, MA: research assistant

    Dante Tipiani: research assistant

    Richard Senzel, MRP: data analyst/programmer

    Sylvan Wallenstein, PhD: statistician

C. Administrative Staff

    Shari Baskin, MPH: administrator

    Matthew Budd, MPA: director of finance

    Christine Rodriguez: administrative assistant

    Tracy Bourne: administrative assistant, billing manager

    Susie West: volunteer

D.   Clinical Characteristics

    1.   Hospital department or division: We are an Institute within the medical school and the Department of Geriatrics and Adult Development.

    2.   Consult Service: Start-up: July 1, 1997

    3.   Dedicated inpatient palliative care unit: 4 beds located on a general medicine teaching unit

    4.   Dedicated inpatient hospice: none

    5.   Home hospice program: affiliate hospice program

    6.   Palliative Care Home Care Program: Mount Sinai's Certified Home Health Agency provides skilled palliative nursing at home, including infusion services.

    7.   Nursing home affiliation: Jewish Home and Hospital

E.   Patient Population, 1999

    1.   New patients per month in the inpatient unit: 7

    2.   New patients per month on the consult service: 36

    3.   Patients per month referred to home care: 12

    4.   Patients per month referred to hospice: 6

    5.   Average inpatient length of stay on the program: 5 days

F. Approximate Funding Sources

   1. Total Program: Approximate Funding Sources FY2000 (includes research and clinical income)

       a. Foundation grants: 32.5%

       b. Federal grants: 20.3%

       c. Endowments: 4.6%

       d. Philanthropy: 20.6%

       e. Hospital support: 1.7%

       f. Medical school support: 2.7%

       g. Physician service income: 7.2%

       h. Other sources: 10.3%

   2. Clinical Program: Approximate Funding Sources FY2000 (excludes research funding)

       a. Philanthropy: 50%

       b. Physician service income: 19%

       c. Hospital support: 16%

       d. Medical school support: 15%

G. Educational Components

   1. Program

       House staff, fellows, and students are educated in the precepts of palliative medicine through bedside teaching, rotations on the Palliative Care Service, and a case-based lecture series. A palliative care rotation is required of all geriatric and hematology–oncology fellows. Many medicine and neurology residents and medical students have chosen palliative care as an elective rotation.

       A short multiple-choice test is administered at the beginning and end of the elective rotation to identify the areas in palliative medicine that residents want to learn about and to tell us whether we are meeting these educational objectives during the rotation. A syllabus of reading is distributed at the start of the rotation.

       An in-service program of interdisciplinary team training in palliative care will be initiated during the year 2000.

2. Trainees

    a. Fellows: All geriatric and hematology–oncology fellows must complete a one-month rotation on the Palliative Care Service.

    b. Residents: Residents can choose a 2–4 week elective rotation.

    c. Medical students: Most commit a certain number of hours over an extended period of time on an elective basis.

    d. Faculty/colleagues: From 1993 to 1996, monthly educational seminars on the legal, medical, and ethical aspects of care at the end of life were held under the Faculty Development Seminars on Ethics and Aging program. In January 1996, a multidepartmental faculty development and education program in palliative medicine and medical ethics was instituted by Drs. Meier, Morrison, and Ahronheim (now at Saint Vincent's Medical Center) and Jane Morris, MS, RN. A new series of monthly seminars on research and methodology in palliative care began in February 2000 under the auspices of the Hertzberg Institute.

III. Research Component: Funding Sources

    A. Federal grants: 36%

    B. Foundation grants: 64%

    C. Industry: none

    D. Intramural: none

MEDIAN AGE: 71 YEARS (18–104 YEARS)

Ethnicity:

48% White

25% African-American

22% Latino

5% Other

Patients' Karnofsky performance status at the time of consult:

18% moribund

33% very sick

27% severely disabled

13% disabled requiring assistance

9% normal activity requiring frequent care

Palliative Care Service diagnoses:

Cancer	54.4%
HIV	7.6%
Dementia	6.8%
Stroke/Coma	6.2%
Cardiac	6.6%
End-stage lung disease	5.7%
End-stage liver disease	4.8%
End-stage renal disease	1.8%
Other	6.1%

Site of discharge or death for palliative care patients:

Died at discharge	51%
Home with hospice	10%
Home with home care	12%
Inpatient hospice	11%
Nursing home	10%
Other	6%

Percentage of palliative care families satisfied or very satisfied with:

Control of pain	95%
Control of other symptoms	92%
Support of patient's quality of life	89%
Support for family stress/anxiety	84%
Manner in which they were told of patient's terminal illness:	88%

Percentage of adult hospital deaths served by Palliative Care Service:

July 1997–April 1999:	14%
May–June 1999:	25%

The Lilian and Benjamin Hertzberg Pallitative
Care Institute, Mount Sinai School of Medicine
Funding Sources FY2000*

Foundation Grants	32%	■
Philanthropy	21%	■
Federal Grants	20%	■
Other Sources	10%	■
Physician Service Income	7%	■
Endowments	5%	■
Medical School Support	3%	■
Hospital Support	2%	■

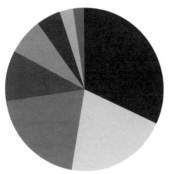

*Includes research and clinical income.

The Lilian and Benjamin Hertzberg Pallitative
Care Institute, Mount Sinai School of Medicine
Clinical Program: Funding Sources*

Philanthropy	50%	■
Physician Service Income	19%	■
Hospital Support	16%	■
Medical School Support	15%	■

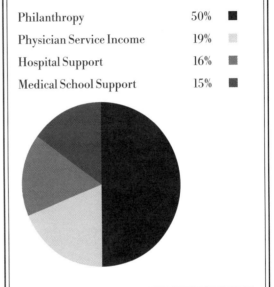

*Excludes research funding.

1. National Institute on Aging (NIH), Academic Career Leadership Award. *Palliative Care and the Elderly*. Principal Investigator: Diane E. Meier, MD. This Geriatric Leadership Academic Award is meant to promote the creation of a strong faculty development program of research and training in palliative medicine and aging at the Mount Sinai School of Medicine. 1999–2004

2. National Institute on Aging (NIH), Mentored Clinical Scientist Development Award. *Pain and Delirium in Hip Fracture Patients*. Principal Investigator: R. Sean Morrison, MD. The purpose of this award is to examine the management of pain and delirium in hip fracture patients. 1998–2003

3. The Robert Wood Johnson Foundation. Center to Advance Palliative Care in Hospitals and Health Systems. Principal Investigators: Christine K. Cassel, MD, and Diane E. Meier, MD. The resource center seeks to foster the development of new hospital and nursing home-based palliative care programs by serving as a clearing house and network. It quantifies and describes existing programs, brings existing organizations together as resources, identifies ways to encourage the development of programs in their early stages, provides expert consultations on program development and staff training, and convenes a process for standard setting for hospital-based palliative care programs. 1999–2003

4. Agency for Health Research and Quality. *Interventions to Improve Pain Outcomes*. Principal Investigator: R. Sean Morrison, MD. This project seeks to develop an institutional model for assessing and treating the pain of seriously ill patients in acute care hospitals.

5. American Federation for Aging Research (AFAR). The Paul Beeson Physician Faculty Scholars in Aging Research Award. *Controlled Trial of Pharmacologic Therapy for Treatment of Delirium in Geriatric Patients*. Principal Investigator: R. Sean Morrison, MD. This research project seeks to examine the management of pain in hip fracture patients and the related problem of delirium.

6. United Hospital Fund. *Community Oriented Palliative Care Network*. Principal Investigator: R. Sean Morrison, MD. The objective is to unite Mount Sinai health system partners with a

network of community-based organizations to provide medical care and support for patients with serious and life-threatening illnesses and for their caregivers.

7. The Robert Wood Johnson Foundation. *Improving End-of-Life Care: Integrating Community Case Management and Palliative Care.* Principal Investigators: Diane E. Meier, MD, and William Thar, MD. The objective is to examine the feasibility of assessing palliative care for patients living at home with feedback to physicians under managed care. 1998–2001

8. The Robert Wood Johnson Foundation. *National Directory of Hospital-Based Palliative Care Programs.* Principal Investigator: Cynthia Pan, MD. The objective is to identify existing and emerging hospital-based palliative care programs and to create a directory of programs in the United States. 1999–2000

9. Intramural Funding. *New York City Opioid Availability Study.* Principal Investigator: R. Sean Morrison, MD. The objective is to gather data regarding the availability of opioids and other pain medications in community pharmacies throughout the five boroughs of New York City. 1999–2000

10. Milbank Memorial Fund. *Perceptions of Financing: Hospital-Based Palliative Care Programs.* Principal Investigator: Christine K. Cassel, MD. The objective is to survey leaders and stakeholders in palliative medicine, hospital administration, and policy experts on a variety of payment and financing issues. 1999–2000

11. Intramural Funding. *Enhancement of Health Care Proxy Awareness.* Principal Investigators: Diane E. Meier, MD, and Stanley Tuhrim, MD. The objective is to increase the number of completed health care proxies among all Mount Sinai physicians and staff. 1999–2000

12. The Stephen and May Cavin Leeman Foundation, The Evelyn Nef Foundation, The Herman Goldman Foundation. *Evaluation of a Hospital-Based Palliative Care Program.* Principal Investigator: Diane E. Meier, MD. The purpose is to expand and refine Mount Sinai's palliative care database and data management system. The generous support of these three foundations has defrayed the cost of this vital part of our research program and information system. 1998–2000

13. The Healthcare Foundation of New Jersey. *A Palliative Care Training Program for Internal Medicine Residents and Fellows.* Principal Investigator: Diane E. Meier, MD. The objective is to create an educational model that promotes integrated clinical expertise in palliative medicine. This program will be offered in collaboration with the major fellowship and residency training programs of the New Jersey affiliates of the Mount Sinai–NYU Health System. The model can be used by other institutions and health care settings. 1999–2001

Palliative Care and Home Hospice Program
Northwestern Memorial Hospital

Charles F. von Gunten

Executive Summary

Northwestern Memorial Hospital (NMH) established its hospice and palliative care program step by step over 17 years. The program has three components: a consultation service, an acute inpatient unit, and a home hospice program. During 1997, the consultation service had an average of 57 new patients per month ranging in age from 45 to 80 years old. During 1996, the 12-bed acute care inpatient unit had an average midnight census of 9.8 patients. That average dropped to 6.9 in 1997, due to new treatments for AIDS, and rose to 9.0 in the third quarter of 1998. The inpatient unit cares for more than one third of all dying patients in Northwestern Memorial, a 779-bed private nonprofit hospital. Patients need not have hospice insurance benefits to be admitted to the acute care unit. The home hospice program serves patients living within the city of Chicago.

In 1997, a total of 800 patients were referred to the program, and 370 of them died. The median length of stay was 31 days. A total of 219 attending physicians cared for patients in the program during the three-year period 1995–1997. Revenues exceeded direct expenses by $1.48 million. That figure excludes physicians' services that were not covered under the Medicare hospice benefit. The group practice that bills for the physicians collected an average of 50.5 percent of its charges over the four years 1994–1997. We conclude that a program of hospice and palliative care can be successful in a private teaching hospital in the United States.

 Inspiration and Motivation

The program at Northwestern evolved over 17 years. The original inspiration for the hospice program came from nurses working at the hospital. When the Joint Commission for Accreditation of Hospitals (JCAH) reviewed the hospital in 1980, it recommended more community outreach. To respond to this recommendation, the hospital developed a supportive care program for patients at home, primarily as an initiative of the Department of Nursing. Two nurses, a social worker, a chaplain, and a medical director staffed the program; they worked as a team and visited terminally ill patients at home. The hospital did not use the term "hospice program" at that time because of objections from the hospital medical staff. Jeanne Martinez, R.N., M.P.H., who was recruited from gynecological oncology to participate in the planning, and who worked as one of the first nurses in the supportive care program, remembers the program as "taking any patients we could—the most difficult discharge problems that no one else wanted."

She also remembers that its medical directors—first a psychiatrist, then a geriatrician—maintained other full-time commitments and that the team therefore lacked enough attention from a committed, knowledgeable physician. This program was the precursor of our current home hospice program.

The next major step in the program's evolution occurred in 1986. Almost simultaneously, the hospital opened a dedicated 10-bed unit and recruited a junior oncologist to spend 25 percent of her time as medical director of the program. This oncologist, Jamie Von Roenn, M.D., was enthusiastic, committed to addressing quality-of-life issues as part of medical oncology, and able to work with an interdisciplinary team.

In 1993, I was recruited to join the faculty and became the medical director of the hospice program. My primary motivations were my experiences caring for patients with cancer during my residency in internal medicine and my fellowship in hematology/oncology, and the mentorship of Dr. Von Roenn and of Dr. Sigmund Weitzman, chief of the Division of Hematology/Oncology. Patients and their families taught me the professional satisfaction of providing care during life-threatening illness. Dr. Von Roenn introduced me to the satisfaction of working with an interdisciplinary team, both in

oncology and in the hospice. A successful academic physician whose professional scope easily spanned the spectrum from diagnosis to death, Dr. Von Roenn became a role model for me. By working with her, and by covering her practice for five months as a first-year fellow while she was on health/maternity leave, I developed a profound working knowledge of how to couple palliative care principles and academic medical oncology. Dr. Weitzman encouraged me to consider an academic career in palliative medicine within his division.

During my fellowship training, in an academic division with 16 physicians on the faculty, I could compare Dr. Von Roenn's practice with that of others in the division. Her approach impressed me. From the initial consultation onward, she incorporated principles of hospice and palliative care—involvement of other disciplines and direct communication and planning with patient and family about the full range of treatments and the possible outcomes, including death. Patients and families were more satisfied, and the bumpy places were much smoother. Some difficulties in communication and choosing treatments that I observed with other faculty were prevented by her practices.

When I became medical director of the hospice program in 1993, I began the consultation service to broaden palliative care so that it would begin earlier in the course of disease than it does in most U.S. hospice programs. Dr. Sigmund Weitzman encouraged me and committed the Division of Hematology/Oncology by making rotation on the consultation service mandatory for the division's fellows. To observe similar programs, I visited Dr. Declan Walsh at the Cleveland Clinic (Goldstein, Walsh, and Horvitz, 1996; Walsh et al., 1994) and doctors at three institutions in London—Nigel Sykes and Mary Baines at St. Christopher's Hospice, Geoff Hanks at St. Thomas' Hospital, and Janet Hardy at the Royal Marsden Hospital. These travels were extraordinarily helpful in crystallizing my plans for an academic palliative care service.

That same year, I polled the hospital's medical staff about their attitudes toward the hospice program, expecting a medium or low overall score. I planned to use this as a baseline against which to measure change after the consultation service began (von Gunten et al., 1995a). Unfortunately or fortunately, the response was so favorable that there was no room for change. More than 90 percent of the physician respondents thought the program was helpful, and more than 95 percent thought it was an important part of the medical center. While there are methodological problems with the study, I think it is safe to say that the hospice and palliative care program is considered integral to the academic center. In light of the medical staff's

reluctance to call the supportive care program "hospice care" in 1980, I think these changes in attitude demonstrate the importance of persistence, leadership, and time in institutionalizing programs in hospitals.

The most rewarding aspect of the program's development has been the collegial relationships that develop around the care of patients—relationships among students, residents, fellows, attending physicians, nurses, people in other medical disciplines, patients, and families. When hospice and palliative care are added to typical hospital medical care, similar outcomes result.

For example, a man with advanced lung cancer was recently admitted to the acute oncology unit with toxicity related to chemotherapy. The attending physician and the house staff perceived him and his family as "in denial" and unrealistic because they demanded additional chemotherapy, total parenteral nutrition, and "answers" from the medical staff. In other words, there was no therapeutic alliance. We introduced hospice and palliative care concepts, not in opposition to, but as part of, his standard oncology care. As a consulting attending, I directed the house staff to assess the patient and family holistically, including their physical, psychological, social, and spiritual needs. I included nurses and other staff members in the assessment and in discussions about treatment plans. I held a family meeting, including the house staff, where we examined both the content and process of the treatment. The outcome was that the patient and family established a therapeutic alliance with their health care team. The medical team gained confidence in approaching the difficult, but common, challenges of inpatient oncology. The nursing staff was happy that cooperation replaced conflict. The administration was happy because a case that could have led to frequent, expensive, futile therapies and frequent hospitalizations was treated more appropriately. That sense of rising to a challenge together and sharing the work is invigorating and gratifying.

 Program Development
. . . .

The program consists of three elements: home hospice care, an acute inpatient unit, and an inpatient consultation service. We manage and finance the elements as a single program, supported by multiple revenue streams from hospice benefits, acute inpatient reimbursement, and fee-for-service professional billing. The infrastructure of a successful, large, nonprofit academic medical center supports the program. Patient-related revenue supports direct expenses of the program. We use philanthropy only to provide "extra" care at home, not to support the program directly.

Home Hospice
The home hospice program began as the supportive care program in 1982. The program became Medicare-certified and accredited by the Joint Commission on Accreditation of Healthcare Organizations (JCAHO) in 1992. As with all such programs, more than 80 percent of the patient-care days are provided in the patient's home. The program controls costs in part by taking advantage of hospital-based rates for drugs and diagnostic tests. Revenue comes from the Medicare Hospice Benefit, Illinois State Medicaid, and commercial payers. In fiscal year 1997, this revenue was 68 percent Medicare, 15 percent Medicaid, and 10 percent commercial insurance. In Illinois, Medicare and Medicaid use the same per diem formula to pay for care. Commercial insurance payments are usually negotiated for each patient, sometimes as a per diem and sometimes as fee-for-service.

Inpatient Unit
Home hospice patients who were admitted to the general hospital often received treatment that was not part of the plan of care chosen by the patient, family, hospice program, and attending physician. Even when the patient and family had chosen hospice care, once patients were admitted to the general hospital, "business as usual" became the driving force. In response, the home hospice

program planned a 10-bed inpatient unit on an existing hospital ward in 1986.

A gift of $250,000 from Cancer Baseball Charities for renovation made it possible to open the unit in 1987. This gift illustrates the adage that chance favors the prepared mind. The baseball charities had decided to make clinical care their priority that year. When their representatives were in the hospital development office, Jeanne Martinez, R.N., M.P.H., the hospice's nurse administrator, happened to be there, too. She promptly suggested the hospice program as the recipient of their gift.

As part of the planning for the inpatient unit, the program was officially named the Hospice Program of Northwestern Memorial Hospital in 1986. This was significant. Attending physicians had initially wanted to avoid the word "hospice." When the unit opened, Dr. Jamie Von Roenn, a newly recruited faculty member in hematology/oncology, became its medical director. Academically, it was connected to the medical school through the Division of Hematology/Oncology in the Department of Medicine. After philanthropy paid the renovation costs, fee-for-service billing for acute care hospitalization provided operating revenues. The unit was not certified or licensed as a hospice unit.

Although the unit was designed for home hospice patients needing hospitalization, only 25 percent of patients on the unit come from home. The majority are transferred from other parts of the hospital. Patients' acute care coverage provides reimbursement.

Consultation Service

In 1993, a consultation service began in the rest of the hospital. Jeanne Martinez, the nurse administrator for the hospice, Dr. Sig Weitzman, chief of hematology/oncology, and I planned the service. We had two goals. The first was to make the methods and insights of hospice care available to the larger hospital community. The second was to provide clinical training for medical students, residents, and fellows. The service achieved both goals. In addition, in the year after the consultation service was instituted, use of the inpatient unit increased 30 percent and the median length of stay in the home hospice program increased from 19 to 38 days.

In 1997, the hospital changed the program's name to the Hospice and Palliative Care program, formally recognizing its increased scope of activities and volume of patients. The program resisted becoming certified for the Medicare Hospice Benefit until 1991 because of the risk that palliative care would be defined by a reimbursement mechanism rather than by the principles of good practice. The hospice program had always been much more "liberal" about medical treatments and approaches than similar community-based programs. A major barrier to the integration of hospice care into mainstream medicine has been the tendency to define appropriate patient care by Medicare's hospice benefit regulations, rather than by the patient's needs. Because our program is supported by both hospice benefits and acute care hospital revenue, and has the advantage of hospital purchasing power, the program has been able to provide "aggressive palliative care," including diagnostic tests and treatments like intravenous infusions, blood transfusions, and antibiotics.

The hospice and palliative care program is working across the continuum of palliative care needs for patients and families, striving to be a component of good medical care, not an alternative to other types of care. In many ways, the program exemplifies the aspirations of the medical center as a whole— appropriate, quality care delivered in local, integrated settings that are best for the patient and family, rather than in a traditional inpatient hospital. This health care is in keeping with the strategic plan of the Northwestern Memorial Corporation, of which NMH is a part.

Institutional Culture
NMH is a private nonprofit hospital with roots in two community-based sectarian hospitals

that merged in 1976. In this private practice environment, physician autonomy and patient satisfaction are valued. The hospital's motto is "an academic medical center where the patient comes first." It has a strong referral base and a healthy bottom line. The payer mix for the hospital is approximately 50 percent Medicare, 30 percent commercial insurance, and 18 percent Medicaid. A small population is uninsured.

Institutional Information
. . . .

Northwestern Memorial Hospital is the principal teaching affiliate hospital of Northwestern University Medical School. It is a 779-bed private, nonprofit hospital located in the center of Chicago. It contains all departments of a general hospital except for pediatrics. The dean of the medical school sits on the NMH board of directors, but the hospital's administration and financing are separate from the university's. In fiscal year 1998, the hospital recorded 38,209 admissions, 5 percent more than the previous fiscal year. This figure includes overnight outpatients and skilled nursing cases. The average length of stay for the hospital as a whole was 4.2 days. There were 698 deaths in the hospital, including the emergency department, in fiscal 1997. The emergency department reported 53,180 visits. The hospital reported 247,316 outpatient registrations and 6,480 births. Nine hospitals are loosely affiliated through the Northwestern Healthcare Network but are autonomous. The hospital has no long-term care affiliates.

Metropolitan Chicago has five medical schools with associated medical centers, more than 60 hospitals, 250 home health agencies, and 65 hospice programs. Most commercial insurance plans for patients who are hospitalized at Northwestern Memorial Hospital are under managed care, mainly in PPO plans that reimburse the hospital and its physicians on a negotiated fee-for-service basis. Less than 10 percent of the business is full-risk capitation.

 Program Characteristics

. . . .

The Palliative Care and Home Hospice Program offers three kinds of service. In the acute general hospital, it provides recommendations and assistance through its consultation service. The inpatient unit provides acute palliative care to patients who are too ill to be cared for in other settings. Finally, the program provides home hospice services either as a sole agency or in cooperation with Northwestern Home Health Care—a home health care agency. Physicians associated with the program may see ambulatory outpatients, although this is not yet a formal part of the program.

Consultation Service

The palliative medicine consultation service, which has been described elsewhere, is staffed by a nurse, an attending physician, and rotating fellows, house staff, and medical students (von Gunten et al., 1998a, Weissman, 1997). Patients are seen anywhere in the hospital at the request of the managing service. Figure 1 shows the number of requests for inpatient consultation for fiscal years 1994 through May 1999. The hospital's fiscal year 1997 runs from September 1, 1996 through August 30, 1997. During fiscal year 1997, an average of 57 consultations was requested each month. Consultations are either called to a team member or transmitted through the hospital computer. On weekdays, the team usually sees the patient within 24 hours of the request. Hematology/oncology fellows, with backup from one of the program's physicians, provide consultations on weekends.

Medical center physicians and staff widely perceive the service as helpful. From the volume of consultations, the varied patients seen, and the number of different referring physicians, it seems clear to us that the consultation service has increased the information and skills available to inpatients and their physicians and, to a lesser degree, to ambulatory outpatients. The visibility of the service mirrors that of the hospital's other consultation services, making palliative care normal and routine.

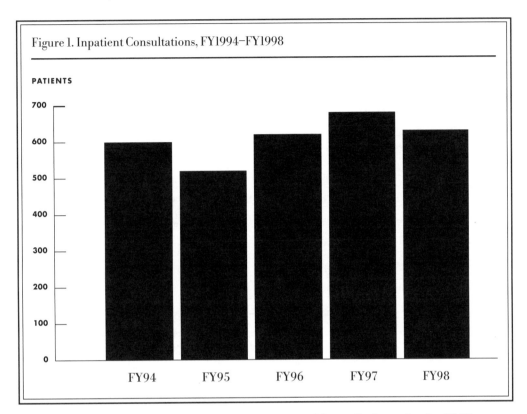

Figure 1. Inpatient Consultations, FY1994–FY1998

PATIENTS

The consultation service does face challenges. It has been difficult to ensure that an attending physician will participate in every consultation in a timely fashion. Reimbursement for nursing has been problematic, like support for specialty nursing in other hospitals. Worse, no specific reimbursement is tied to nurses' work. The palliative consultation nurse is paid from the budget of the inpatient unit. In addition, consultation services are needed, but not provided, to major areas of the medical center, such as cardiology, surgery, renal, pulmonary, and gynecological oncology, or to other parts of the medical complex that NMH belongs to, such as the Veterans Affairs Hospital and the Rehabilitation Institute of Chicago. Most of the nine other hospitals associated with NMH through the Northwestern Healthcare Network also lack consultation services.

These are obvious opportunities for increased growth of the service. Ambulatory outpatients could also benefit from it, particularly AIDS, geriatrics, and cardiology patients. However, growth will require increased support from both the hospital and the medical school.

Acute Inpatient Palliative Care Unit
The inpatient unit consists of 10 acute care beds in large private rooms on a dedicated nursing unit in the hospital (Kellar et al., 1996; Ng and von Gunten, 2000). We plan to add five more beds. Figure 2 shows the average inpatient census at midnight. The midnight census is the count of patients who are alive at midnight in a bed on the unit. Patients who died or were discharged before midnight or who were admitted after midnight are not counted in it. Consequently, up to 16 patients may come through the unit during 24 hours even though the midnight census lists only eight patients for that day. Although this convention for measuring occupancy understates the unit's overall workload, the convention is still widely used by hospitals for reporting and billing purposes. The 43 percent increase in the average census for fiscal year 1994 results from the institution of the consultation service. In fact, the number of inpatient beds was increased from 10 to 12 in 1995 in order to accommodate the increased demand. The drop in the census for fiscal year 1997 is related to the introduction of protease inhibitors in the treatment of AIDS. In 1994 almost 25 percent of our patients had a

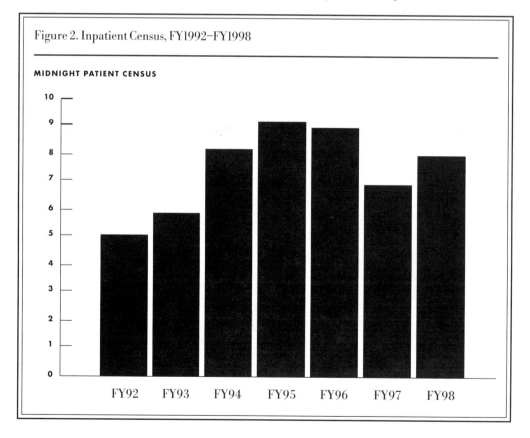

Figure 2. Inpatient Census, FY1992–FY1998

MIDNIGHT PATIENT CENSUS

primary diagnosis of AIDS; in 1997 only 7 percent had AIDS.

Of the 459 patients hospitalized on the unit in fiscal year 1996, 54 percent had Medicare, 13 percent had Medicaid or expected to obtain Medicaid, and 33 percent had commercial insurance. Of those with commercial insurance, less than 10 percent were in an HMO. Virtually all the rest had PPO indemnity plans. Only two patients were uninsured. This breakdown of payments is essentially the same as for patients seen by the consultation service, and for the entire hospital.

In May 1999, the acute inpatient palliative care unit moved into a new building with all other patient care units. Interestingly, the new hospital incorporates many design elements of the old palliative care unit. All patients' rooms in the hospital are private. Except for the intensive care units, all rooms are large and have a foldout couch where a family member can spend the night. Visiting hours on the inpatient palliative care unit are unrestricted. Pets may visit. Full-time professional staff and hospice-trained volunteers are on hand. Some professional staff and volunteers are shared with the home hospice program. For example, the bereavement coordinator works with all families of those who die either on the unit or at home. The full range of services and treatments customarily available in an acute hospital are available. The only requirements for admission

are a do-not-resuscitate order and a choice of primarily palliative treatment. Patients can be admitted direct from homes or doctors' offices at all hours, without being evaluated in the emergency department. Enrollment in a home hospice program is not required.

Patients, families, and physicians are highly satisfied with the palliative inpatient unit, to judge from cards and letters sent to the chief executive officer and from annual surveys, in which patients and families rank the unit's care as among the best in the hospital. Surveys of attending physicians rank the unit's nursing care among the best in the institution.

All insurers and third-party payers that cover hospitalization at NMH cover hospitalization on the palliative inpatient unit. Patients need not have accessed hospice insurance benefits to be admitted. The appropriateness of admissions and continued stays are evaluated with the same criteria as for other patients in the hospital (ISD-AC Criteria, 1996). Despite changes in guidelines for overall use, the denial rate for inpatient charges remains among the lowest in the hospital.

However, the utilization review department has to negotiate and defend the admission of patients to the unit. In one case, a 43-year-old patient with commercial insurance had advanced malignant melanoma. The patient's insurer pays the hospital a negotiated per diem for all of its beneficiaries—about $1,000–$1,600 per day—and certifies utilization based on the severity of illness and the intensity of service (ISD-AC Criteria, 1996). This patient was admitted to the general hospital for fatigue, anemia, fever, and pain. After a palliative medicine consultation, we moved him to the inpatient palliative care unit where the focus was on managing pain, helping his wife and young children cope, and preparing for a safe discharge. The insurer denied the hospital's claim for the five days the patient spent on the unit. The hospital's utilization review department appealed. The insurer denied payment again. The medical director assisted in a second appeal. Finally the insurer paid the full claim.

The inpatient unit makes acute palliative care available to many more patients than a licensed hospice unit could. The flexibility and capacity for high acuity permit this. Yet the inpatient unit, like the consulting service, confronts several challenges. Inadequate education of medical center staff members about the unit's purpose and work persists; many think the unit is a lower-level acuity unit where only terminal care is administered. In addition, the high acuity, complexity, and volume of patients and families, and the frequent deaths, create unique stress for the

unit's staff. The 10-bed unit handles over one third of all in-hospital deaths at NMH.

The confusion of insurers and third-party payers about the difference between the acute unit and inpatient hospice units in the Chicago area creates tension and extra work for the staff. The unit is an acute care unit. Insurers consider inpatient hospices as only skilled-care units. The confusion of third-party payers is exacerbated because the tools that utilization review personnel employ ignore all medical care that could even vaguely be construed as palliative. Consequently, the hospital's utilization review department and the staff of the program endure considerable stress while working with case managers to describe the needs and care of patient after patient after patient.

The program does not supply skilled care for patients needing hospice and palliative care. It would be helpful to provide this care for patients who do not need acute care but cannot be cared for in a nursing home or their own homes. However, the state of Illinois requires a certificate of need for skilled care beds, and there is a moratorium on new beds. In addition, acute care reimbursement has been obtained for patients despite the utilization review battles. For those few patients who stay on the unit for an extended period, skilled care rates are sometimes negotiated. There is no provision for residential hospice care anywhere in the state of Illinois.

Home Hospice Program

Medicare and the Joint Commission on Accreditation of Healthcare Organizations (JCAHO) certify the home hospice program. The team delivers hospice care to patients and families living within Chicago's city limits. The average census fluctuates between 30 and 50 patients per day. In fiscal year 1997, the program cared for 198 patients at home. Figure 3 summarizes their length of stay. The median length of stay is 31 days with an average of 73.9 days, up from a median of 19 days in 1993 because the consultation service began. Payer sources for 125 patients cared for at home in fiscal year 1997 were 68 percent Medicare, 15 percent public aid, and 10 percent commercial insurance. Six percent of patients at home were uninsured. The program uses the NMH indigent care budget to provide basic hospice care at home, like that provided by the Medicare Hospice Benefit, without regard to the patient's financial situation. Further, the program uses philanthropy to provide care that would otherwise be unavailable—principally the hiring of caregivers for patients who live alone or whose caregivers are frail or working outside the home. We do not use philanthropy for basic hospice care that the NMH indigent budget covers. The indigent

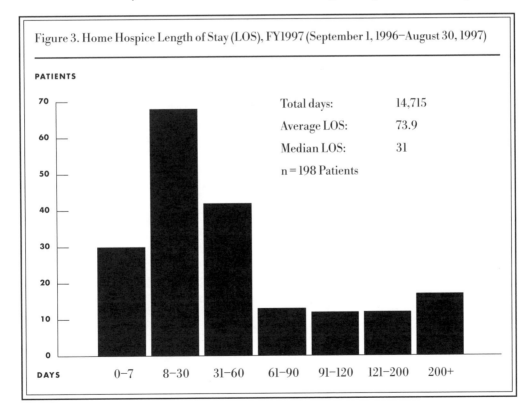

Figure 3. Home Hospice Length of Stay (LOS), FY1997 (September 1, 1996–August 30, 1997)

PATIENTS

Total days: 14,715
Average LOS: 73.9
Median LOS: 31
n = 198 Patients

DAYS   0–7   8–30   31–60   61–90   91–120   121–200   200+

budget accounts for less than 2 percent of hospital expenses.

As with other home hospice programs, the program prevents unnecessary admissions to acute hospital and skilled nursing facilities and avoids unnecessary use of the emergency department. Nurses are on call 24 hours a day, seven days a week to respond rapidly when symptoms change. The program works flexibly to coordinate care with Northwestern Home Health Agency, a separate company owned by the hospital corporation to maximize patient benefit by permitting access to additional services, such as home infusion therapy.

We have found that patient and family satisfaction with the home hospice program is extremely high. However, the program has difficulty finding resources to care for the many patients who live alone so that they are safe in the location they prefer. Some patients live in areas with high crime rates where armed guards must accompany staff members and where it is unsafe for the staff to travel at all at certain times. Some patients have high-tech care needs or receive therapies that have both life-prolonging and palliative purposes that are not easily accommodated by conventional hospice insurance benefits. As NMH is both a community hospital and a tertiary-care referral center, some patients in the consultation or inpatient parts of the program live outside the NMH home

hospice service area. In those cases, our program facilitates referrals to other hospice programs.

Program Operations

Figure 4 shows the total number of referrals, including inpatient consultations, and the total number of patients who died as inpatients or at home. The opening of the inpatient unit in 1987 nearly doubled of the number of patients and families the program served. The introduction of the consultation service in 1993 induced another 30 percent increase in volume.

Diagnoses for patients seen by the program have changed. In 1982, nearly all patients had cancer. By 1994, 56 percent of patients had cancer, 26 percent had AIDS, and 18 percent had other noncancer diagnoses. However, the introduction of protease inhibitors in 1995 changed the demographics. In 1997, 71 percent of patients had cancer, 7 percent had AIDS, and 22 percent had other noncancer diagnoses.

The program has had a marked effect on the location of patients' deaths. Total deaths in the hospital, including those in the emergency department, have remained remarkably constant at approximately 700 patients per year since 1990, despite an increase in admissions of approximately 6 percent per year. From 1990 to 1998 the

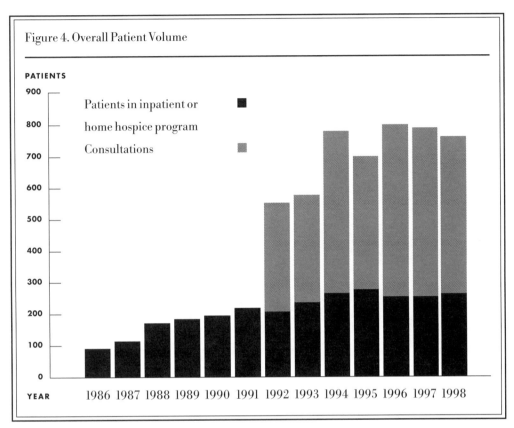

Figure 4. Overall Patient Volume

PATIENTS

Patients in inpatient or home hospice program ■

Consultations ■

YEAR 1986 1987 1988 1989 1990 1991 1992 1993 1994 1995 1996 1997 1998

percentage of people dying in the intensive care units, operating rooms, and emergency department has remained at approximately 40 percent of all deaths. However, by 1995, two years after the consultation service started, the percentage of patients dying in the inpatient palliative care unit rose from 25 to 38 percent, with a corresponding decrease on the general medical/surgical units. During the six months ending May 1999, there were only 18 deaths on the inpatient oncology unit. Better palliative care on a dedicated unit, and more appropriate use of health care resources there, have had a large

effect on the care of the dying in the hospital.

Despite its being a teaching hospital, NMH is a private hospital whose medical staff is approximately half full-time faculty and half private practitioners. Patients are admitted to the hospital, and to the home hospice program, under the aegis of the patient's primary attending physician. During the three years from fiscal year 1994 through fiscal year 1997, 219 physicians referred 2,100 patients to the program. More than half of those 219 physicians were general internists. (There are no family physicians on staff at the hospital.) Only 14

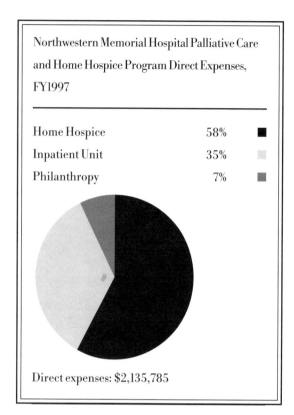

Northwestern Memorial Hospital Palliative Care and Home Hospice Program Direct Expenses, FY1997

Home Hospice	58%	■
Inpatient Unit	35%	▨
Philanthropy	7%	■

Direct expenses: $2,135,785

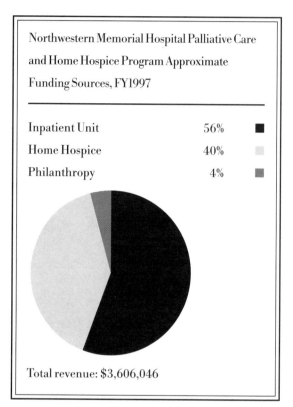

Northwestern Memorial Hospital Palliative Care and Home Hospice Program Approximate Funding Sources, FY1997

Inpatient Unit	56%	■
Home Hospice	40%	▨
Philanthropy	4%	■

Total revenue: $3,606,046

percent of the 219 were oncologists. Nine percent of them were surgeons. This is evidence of the broad acceptance and integration of the program into the culture of the medical center (von Gunten, 1995a).

The pie charts show total revenue and direct expenses for the program in fiscal year 1997. Indirect expenses are not shown. These revenue figures do not include physicians' fee-for-service billing for services not covered by the Medicare Hospice Benefit. Table 1 shows personnel who are supported as direct expenses from the indicated revenue. Philanthropy that pays for uncovered home hospice services has helped

patients like an elderly woman with pancreatic cancer who lived in a rented apartment on the south side of Chicago. Her children lived in other cities. She wanted to die at home but had no primary caregiver. Medicare's hospice benefit does not cover attendant care beyond 12 hours a week. We used our program's philanthropic funds to hire a nurse's aide around the clock for 60 days so that the patient could remain safely at home.

One full-time and one part-time faculty physician staff the program with the assistance of three private practice physicians from the community. The

Table 1: Personnel Supported by Clinical Revenue, Fiscal Year 1997

1	Nurse Administrator
1	Medical (0.25 FTE [full-time equivalent])
1	Hospice Physician (0.2 FTE)
2	Nurse Home-Hospice Care Coordinators
12	Inpatient Nurses
6	Home Hospice Nurses
2	Social Workers
1	Chaplain
2	Home Nursing Aides
1	Volunteer Coordinator
1	Bereavement Coordinator
1	Computer Systems Coordinator
2	Secretaries

charges $296. Commercial payers will reimburse about $250. Medicare pays only $90, and Medicaid pays $30. Clearly, the proportion of patients in each category affects overall reimbursement.

Educational Component

I have described educational programs based in this clinical program elsewhere (von Gunten et al., 1994; von Gunten et al., 1995b; von Gunten et al., 1998b). Fellows in hematology/oncology and in geriatrics are required to rotate for a month. Residents in internal medicine and psychiatry rotate on an elective basis. Medical students learn about the program as an elective in their fourth year or through required course work in their first two years. Numerous students, residents, and practicing physicians rotate for varying periods, as nursing and social work students do.

collection rate for these bills by the Northwestern Medical Faculty Foundation (NMFF, the faculty group practice) averaged 50.5 percent from 1993 to 1997. This compares with a collection rate of approximately 58 percent for the entire hematology/oncology division. Similar information is not available to us from other divisions in NMFF. My analysis suggests that the difference between 50.5 and 58 percent stems from a higher proportion of Medicare patients on the Hospice/Palliative Care Service than in general hematology/ oncology. For example, for a high-complexity physician code, the faculty foundation

% EFFORT

1R25CA66933-01A2   9/1/96–6/30/99   10%

NIH/NCI   Total Direct Cost $218,865

Clinical Elective in Hospice/Palliative Medicine for House Staff

Primary investigator: Charles F. von Gunten, MD, PhD

Curriculum development and evaluation for residents training in general internal medicine.

2R25CA66771-04   9/30/94–9/29/00   5%

NIH/NCI   Total Direct Cost $202,737

Physician Hospice/Palliative Care Training: UNIPACS

PI: Porter Storey, MD

Create and evaluate self-teaching modules in palliative medicine for physicians. Dr. von Gunten is involved in writing the Unipac on AIDS.

NIH/NCI   12/01/98–11/30/00

Dying, Death and Grief: Internet Project Total Direct Cost $202,651

PI: Sara Knight

A continuing education effort for physicians and other health care providers.

Robert Wood Johnson Foundation   1/1/98–12/31/00   15%

Residency Training in End-of-Life Care   Total Direct Cost $164,163

PI: David Weissman, MD

A faculty development program to help residency programs across the country incorporate palliative care education into their training programs.

Center for Palliative Medicine Education & Research   10/1/95–9/30/97

AV Davis Foundations   Total Direct Cost $200,000

Established the center. Supports a nurse coordinator and visiting fellows. Funding for visiting fellows continues beyond the original funding period.

Roxane Visiting Scholars Program | 7/1/95–continuing

Roxane Laboratories, Inc. | Total Direct Cost $146,000

Provides support for physicians and other health care providers to visit for one week as a "mini-internship."

Robert Wood Johnson Foundation | 1/1/96–5/31/99 | 60%

Education for Physicians in End-of-Life Care | Total Direct Cost $1,500,000

PI: Linda Emanuel, MD, PhD

Develop and disseminate a curriculum with basic skills for U.S. physicians.

Robert Wood Johnson Foundation | 6/1/99–5/31/00 | 25%

Education for Physicians in End-of-Life Care | Total Direct Cost $400,000

PI: Linda Emanuel, MD, PhD

Develop and disseminate a curriculum with basic skills for U.S. physicians.

R25CA57818-04 | 7/1/94–6/31/97 | 10%

NIH/NCI | Total Direct Cost: $270,640

Cancer Pain Education–An Analgesic Dosing Service

PI: Charles von Gunten, MD, PhD

A novel approach to the education of house staff regarding cancer pain management.

Open Society Institute | 7/1/95–6/39/98 | 60%

Project on Death in America | Total Direct Cost $225,000

Soros Faculty Scholar

A faculty development grant for Dr. von Gunten to further his development as a leader in U.S. palliative care.

Hospice of the Texas Medical Center

Mexiletine for Neuropathic Pain

PI: Charles von Gunten, MD, PhD

A phase II placebo-controlled trial of mexiletine for cancer-related neuropathic pain.

Anesta Corporation

Oral Fentanyl for Cancer Breakthrough Pain

PI: Charles von Gunten, MD, PhD

A phase II placebo-controlled trial of oral fentanyl for cancer breakthrough pain.

Purdue Pharma, Inc.

Sustained-Release Hydromorphone for Cancer Pain

PI: Charles von Gunten, MD, PhD

A Phase II placebo-controlled trial of oral hydromorphone for cancer pain.

REFERENCES

Goldstein, P., D. Walsh, and L.U. Horvitz. 1996. The Cleveland Clinic Foundation Harry R. Horvitz Palliative Care Center. *Support Care in Cancer*, 4:329-33.

ISD-AC Criteria (Adult) Pocket Version 1996: Intensity of Service, Severity of Illness, and Discharge Screens for Acute Care. InterQual: North Hampton, N.H.

Kellar, N., J. Martinez, N. Finis, A. Bolger, and C.F. von Gunten. 1996. Characterization of an Acute Inpatient Hospice Palliative Care Unit in a U.S. Teaching Hospital. *Journal of Nursing Administration*, 26:16-20.

Ng, K., and C. von Gunten. 2000. Symptoms and Attitudes of 100 Consecutive Patients Admitted to an Acute Hospice/Palliative Care Unit. *Journal of Pain and Symptom Management*, in press.

von Gunten, C.F., S. Weitzman, and J.H. Von Roenn. 1994. Housestaff Training in Cancer Pain Education. *Journal of Cancer Education*, 9:230-4.

von Gunten, C.F., J.H. Von Roenn, K.J. Neely, J. Martinez, and S. Weitzman. 1995a. Hospice and Palliative Care: Evaluation of the Attitudes and Practices of the Physician Faculty of an Academic Hospital. *American Journal of Hospice and Palliative Care*, 12(4):38-42.

von Gunten, C.F., J.H. Von Roenn, W. Gradishar, and S. Weitzman. 1995b. Hospice/Palliative Medicine Rotation for Fellows Training in Hematology/Oncology. *Journal of Cancer Education*, 10:200-3.

von Gunten, C.F., B. Camden, K.J. Neely, G. Franz, and J. Martinez. 1998a. Prospective Evaluation of Referrals to a Hospice/Palliative Medicine Consultation Service. *Journal of Palliative Medicine*, 1(1):45-53.

von Gunten, C.F., J. Martinez, K.J. Neely, M. Twaddle, and M. Preodor. 1998b. Clinical Experience in Hospice and Palliative Medicine for Clinicians in Practice. *Journal of Palliative Medicine*, 1(3):249-55.

Walsh, D., W.R. Gombeski, Jr., P. Goldstein, D. Hayes, and M. Armour. 1994. Managing a Palliative Oncology Program: The Role of a Business Plan. *Journal of Pain and Symptom Management*, 9:109-18.

Weissman, D. 1997. Consultation in Palliative Medicine. *Archives of Internal Medicine*, 157:733-7.

Comprehensive Palliative Care Service
University of Pittsburgh–UPMC

Robert M. Arnold

Executive Summary

The Comprehensive Palliative Care Service began with my personal commitment to caring for dying patients, and with my recognition that care at the end of life and communication among physicians, patients, and families about end-of-life issues needed to be improved. Early in my fellowship from the Project on Death in America (PDIA), I met with oncology nurses and physicians, chaplains, geriatricians, doctors of pharmacy, social workers, representatives from volunteer services, critical-care medicine physicians, and internists representing two hospitals at the University of Pittsburgh Medical Center—UPMC-Presbyterian and UPMC-Shadyside. I found that a number of seemingly unrelated services involving end-of-life care existed within UPMC, including ethics consultation, hospice, and pain management services. More important, I found a group of like-minded individuals with a strong interest in improving palliative care through the development of a Comprehensive Palliative Care Service.

After obtaining information about palliative care programs elsewhere, we decided to use a model similar to Northwestern University's program, a hospital-based consultation service that emphasizes family support along with patient care and is integrated with ambulatory and home-based programs. Armed with data collected from several surveys, we eventually obtained support from key individuals at UPMC. Funding was provided for one full-time nurse practitioner, a half-time physician for performing consults (minus the amount we brought in through billing), and a half-time secretary. Other staff members either volunteer their services or are paid by their respective departments.

Consultations are available seven days a week, 24 hours a day. Attending physicians or the house staff, with the attending physician's permission, can request a consultation. The Service contacts the patient's attending physician or the house staff within two hours of their request to determine the consultation's goals. The Service reviews all

Acknowledgments: I thank the wonderful group with which I have had the pleasure to work and the patients and families who have taught us so much. Comments from Richard Simmons, Wishwa Kapoor, Mary Ellen Cowan, David Barnard, and Ellen Redinbaugh improved the report. Deborah L. Seltzer provided editorial input.

Support: Dr. Arnold received support from the Greenwall Foundation, the Open Society's Project on Death in America Faculty Scholars Program, Ladies Hospital Aid Society of Western Pennsylvania, and LAS Trust Foundation.

pathology and radiology studies, interviews and examines the patient, and meets with the family before making its recommendations. To facilitate our evaluation, we developed intake forms for the patient and family. Both the palliative care attending and the nurse practitioner see the patient within 24 hours of the request. They then make referrals to appropriate members of the palliative care team, including a psychologist, a doctor of pharmacy with special expertise in pain management, a wound care nurse, a spiritual counselor, and a primary social worker.

We provide three grief and bereavement programs for patients: a follow-up program for patients who are still alive; a bereavement program for families of patients who have died in the hospital; and a family support program for families of critically ill patients admitted to the ICU. In addition we put together a team to provide staff bereavement rounds, to offer psychosocial support for health care providers who are grieving over patient losses.

Education plays a central role in the Comprehensive Palliative Care Service in four ways. We train nurses on two units in the hospital to provide better palliative care; we opened the consult service to medical students, residents, fellows, and nurse practitioners to improve their palliative care skills; we train medical students and house staff in palliative care; and we develop

training for many other residency programs inside and outside of UPMC.

To continue its work the Service seeks visibility by meeting with groups of attendings, nurses, and house staff and meeting individually with physicians who admit a large number of patients to the hospital. The Service maintains strong institutional ties through monthly reports to, and quarterly meetings with, institutional leaders. To evaluate our work, we periodically survey attendings, house staff, nurses, social workers, patients, and families.

There were obstacles to developing the Service. Initially, when the Section for Palliative Care and Medical Ethics was established within the Division of General Internal Medicine to house the Service, the Director of the Center for Bioethics and Health Law was concerned that the Section was designed as a competitor; fortunately, we were able to alleviate his concerns. Administratively, the structure of the Service is complex. It is funded by the Institute of Performance Improvement and operated through General Internal Medicine with volunteers and consultants from many departments within UPMC. Personnel report to different managers, and thus their responsibilities have to be negotiated carefully.

Fiscal issues are also complex. Physicians' services are billed as consultations, and it has been difficult to determine our billable income. There were large differences in billing by different physicians. We are working with the billing department to develop standards for billing. We have learned that it is critical to ensure at the outset that physicians and other staff members share a common understanding of the goals of the Service and the time it requires. One obstacle was an unintentional slighting of UPMC's social workers. Since much of our work involves tasks that they traditionally performed, we should have spent more time communicating with them during the development of the program. Finally, we have had some difficulty in obtaining consults from UPMC-Shadyside, a private hospital that had recently merged with UPMC.

The Comprehensive Palliative Care Service has grown significantly and has made tremendous strides in improving the care of terminally ill patients and their families.

 Inspiration and Motivation
. . . .

For many years, my primary medical work focused on caring for patients who were HIV seropositive. At that time, there were no anti-retrovirals, and the care of these patients was largely palliative. Unlike many physicians, I found that I enjoyed caring for dying patients. The quality of our relationships seemed different from those I developed with other patients. In a short time, I was able to

talk with these patients about their hopes and concerns. This led to a deep bond between us and a commitment on my part to make the rest of their lives as rich as possible. I learned that even when death was inevitable, I could do a lot to improve the quality of a patient's life. I began to derive satisfaction from being able to decrease patients' symptoms and provide them with a couple of extra weeks at home with their families.

I learned a great deal from these patients. I learned about the importance of relationships, about the different ways that people obtain meaning from their daily routines, about different ways to say good-bye, and about the variety of ways in which people grapple with the existential dimensions of life. Caring for dying patients also taught me much about the power of language and about my own unexamined assumptions about what it means to be a doctor. After one patient angrily corrected me, I stopped talking about patients "failing" their chemotherapy. Nor do I talk about comfort measures *only* or compare aggressive treatments to palliative care.

My burgeoning practice in end-of-life care focused my scholarly interest in bioethics and communication skills. I began to study how doctors could communicate more effectively about advance planning. In 1996, I decided to pursue these interests by applying for a fellowship from the Project on

Death in America. I proposed to train a select group of geriatricians, oncologists, and HIV doctors to teach other physicians to communicate more effectively regarding the ethical, psychosocial, and existential issues surrounding end-of-life care. Luckily, the grant was funded.

I cannot overestimate the importance of this grant. First, it allowed me to give up my non–palliative care responsibilities. I was able to decrease my case load in general internal medicine and relinquish administrative responsibilities for developing ambulatory care rotations for approximately 60 house staff. Second, the fellowship gave me instant visibility and credibility within the university and the Department of Medicine. Departmental and university newsletters publicized news of the scholarship. Suddenly colleagues viewed me as someone with a national reputation in palliative care.

Third, as a Project on Death in America fellow, I met and communicated with a number of individuals who shared similar interests and had much greater expertise. The first group of scholars—David Weissman, Andrew Billings, and Charles von Gunten—shared their experiences regarding palliative care consultations. They described the clinical, educational, and research value of such a service and encouraged me to consider developing one.

Previous Efforts in Palliative Care

I began meeting with individuals at the University of Pittsburgh Medical Center (UPMC) to determine what others inside the institution were doing in palliative care. I met with oncology nurses and physicians, chaplains, geriatricians, doctors of pharmacy, social workers, representatives from volunteer services, critical-care physicians, and internists. These individuals represented two UPMC hospitals: UPMC-Presbyterian and UPMC-Shadyside. A number of unrelated programs at UPMC were already trying to improve end-of-life care. Both hospitals have ethics committees; the committee at UPMC-Presbyterian is one of the oldest in the country and has a longstanding interest in end-of-life care. UPMC-Presbyterian developed one of the nation's first hospital policies on foregoing life-sustaining treatment. The ethics committee is intimately affiliated with the Center for Bioethics and Health Law and performs approximately 60 ethics consultations each year, most of which deal with end-of-life issues. The UPMC-Shadyside ethics committee, while younger, also has a consultative service and is quite involved in teaching.

The University of Pittsburgh Cancer Institute (UPCI), which has no formal palliative care program, devotes much attention to end-of-life care. UPCI has a pain service managed by a doctor of pharmacy with a national reputation in pain management. She makes daily rounds with the doctors and serves as a resource for the oncologists. The oncology social workers have a great interest in palliative care and have developed family support and bereavement groups in the past.

Six months before our Palliative Care Service was started, the home-based component of UPMC Health System began a hospice program. Pittsburgh's other major health care system had a large and successful hospice program, and the hospital administration viewed UPMC's lack of such a program as a problem. UPMC hired an oncologist and a geriatrician who had worked at a hospice in Cleveland as co-directors of the new hospice. These events were completely independent of my efforts to develop the consulting service; I was unaware of the events at the time. About two years before our Service was instituted, the nurse administrator at UPCI had developed a proposal to create an inpatient, 16-bed hospice. The proposal was unsuccessful. It was considered expensive and it came at a time when the hospital, threatened by the unpredictability of managed care, was intent on transferring patients out of the hospital to alternative settings. Hospital-based palliative care seemed a fiscal impossibility. Similarly, about a year before my own proposal was written, UPCI had tried unsuccessfully to recruit a physician who had completed a

pain fellowship and was interested in palliative care.

Palliative Care Study Group

As I met with interested parties at UPMC, I found that they were eager to expand their efforts in palliative care. They felt—and I agreed—that the time had come to combine the various programs and to determine whether we could build a more comprehensive one. These individuals were from all disciplines—ranging from the volunteer service to the head of the quality assurance committee to a nurse practitioner on the oncology service. The doctor of pharmacy who ran the UPCI pain program, social workers with a great deal of experience in end-of-life care, and the medical directors of the UPMC hospice were also interested in developing a comprehensive program. Within three weeks of the group's initiation, a group of about 20 people began meeting to identify palliative care goals, the means through which to achieve them, and the availability of resources at the UPMC Health System. We met every other Friday at 7:00 A.M. Despite the early hour and participants' busy schedules, attendance remained at 85 to 90 percent for all of our meetings.

We decided that it was important for the new Service to integrate inpatient and outpatient consulting and dedicated inpatient beds. Interestingly, each participating group believed that the Service would be most helpful for other participants. The oncologist believed that while oncologists might consult such a service, the surgeons and general internists would benefit greatly from it. The transplant service reported that they did a good job caring for terminally ill patients but that the oncologists would benefit. The doctors thought the Service would improve the nurses' ability to treat pain, while nurses thought we could help the doctors talk more honestly about dying.

To learn more about setting up a palliative care service, I obtained information from the Cleveland Clinic, Massachusetts General Hospital, Mount Sinai Medical Center, Penn State University, and Northwestern University. This information allowed me to see how other programs had been developed and to understand the financial issues they confronted. We also obtained each program's patient-care assessment forms and referred to them when we developed our own.

We modeled our program most closely on Northwestern University's palliative care program. It has built a very successful hospital-based consultative service and has also developed a horizontally integrated program with ambulatory and home-based services. Northwestern's philosophy of attending to the physical and psychosocial needs of the family, as well as those of the patient, fit into our ideal. Dr. Charles von Gunten, then the director of the Northwestern program, was a great support. He spoke with me often by phone about the political and financial issues involved in starting a program. He also spent a day in Chicago showing a colleague and me around his program and helping us think about how we could start the program in Pittsburgh.

Needs Assessment

To obtain financial and institutional support, we needed data about how patients died at UPMC-Presbyterian Hospital. We conducted various surveys to document the need for our program. Dr. Ann Fraker, a resident at UPMC-Presbyterian, identified 167 patients who had died in January and February of 1996 and examined the effects of advance directives on CPR and other variables associated with terminal care at the hospital. A DNR order was placed on the chart within 48 hours 43 percent of the time. Patients with DNR orders had shorter stays than those who did not (11 days vs. 17 days). Of the 30 patients who had a cardiac arrest without a DNR order, 17 died during the arrest and 13 died in an ICU after having a DNR order placed.

To find out more about patients who might be referred to a palliative care service, we asked the UPMC-Presbyterian house staff and social workers to identify patients whom a palliative consultation might help. Over a two-week period in mid-October 1997, the house staff identified 34 such patients; the social workers identified 35 patients. (Seventeen were identified by both the residents and the social workers). Only one-third of the patients were on the oncology unit. Patients were identified on thoracic surgery, urology, gastrointestinal surgery, trauma/neurology, and neurosurgery units. Fifty-eight percent of the patients identified had Medicare insurance, 33 percent had private insurance, and 9 percent had Medicaid. These patients stayed in the hospital an average of 14.2 days—more than twice as long as the average hospital patient. Approximately 20 percent of them died in the hospital.

At UPMC-Shadyside Hospital we randomly reviewed 25 charts using a "quality of dying" instrument developed by Joan Temo and Joanne Lynn (www.chcr.brown.edu/pcoc/toolkit.htm). As our previous survey regarding DNR orders had found, most decisions regarding life-sustaining treatment were made the day before the patient died. Less than 24 hours before death, most patients were still receiving treatment that might not have been consistent with palliative care. (Ten received IV antibiotics, nine had nasogastric tubes, 22 received IV fluids, 10 had X-rays, and all but one had blood drawn.) Chart reviews revealed that on the day of death and the day before death, symptoms were assessed in less than half of the cases. The charts documented emotional or social support in only 12 of 25 cases, and spiritual support in only eight of the 25. There was no indication of any referral or counseling for bereavement.

Key Supporters

Armed with these data, we approached a number of leaders at UPMC-Presbyterian and UPMC-Shadyside to gain backing for the Palliative Care Service. The Division of Oncology was quite receptive. We had previously negotiated with a co-director of the hospice, who had been involved as a participant in my grant from the Project on Death in America; he was willing to become a consultant to the new service. The doctor of pharmacy in charge of the UPCI pain program was very supportive; she agreed to serve as a pharmacological resource. The Division of Oncology, which had neither time nor resources to fund its own palliative program, saw this as a chance to improve its patient care.

The Division of Geriatrics was similarly supportive. The other co-director of the hospice agreed to serve as the third physician on the consultative service. Both he and the director of the Division of Geriatrics had been involved as participants in my PDIA proposal. In light of their experience caring for elderly dying patients in the hospital, they were convinced that a palliative care service would prove valuable.

My supervisor, Wishwa Kapoor, the chief of the Division of General Internal Medicine, was supportive as well. His major concern was that the division receive credit and have administrative responsibility for the new program. Given the multidisciplinary character of the program and the fact that our faculty came from many divisions and departments, it would have made the most sense to start a Center of Palliative Care. However, this is administratively and politically difficult and requires a fair amount of money. As an interim step, and one that allowed me to retain control of the program, we developed a Section of Palliative Care and Medical Ethics within the Division of General Internal Medicine.

This action caused concern at the Center for Bioethics and Health Law. The Center had been created about 15 years earlier to promote teaching and research in medical ethics within the university, particularly the health science center. The Center has been very successful and has developed a nationally recognized program for teaching medical students, as well as strong research programs on end-on-life care, organ donation, and informed consent. I was, and still am, the associate director of education for the Center. There was concern

that a separate Section of Palliative Care and Medical Ethics within the Department of Medicine would fragment the Center's efforts and the University's resources for medical ethics. We did not want to build a competing program. Our focus was on palliative care, rather than on medical ethics in general. (In fact, the reason we included "Medical Ethics" in the title of the Section had more to do with supporting members of the Center of Bioethics and Health Law whose primary academic appointments were in General Internal Medicine than with anything else.) I spoke with Alan Meisel, director of the Center, about these issues and allayed his fears.

While many individuals were supportive, none could provide financial support. I therefore went to Dr. Richard Simmons, the medical director of the UPMC Health System and the director of the Institute for Performance Improvement and the previous chair of the Department of Surgery. In these capacities, Dr. Simmons has a great deal of influence with doctors and administrators within the institution. Dr. Simmons agreed with my views of the importance of this program and was willing to pursue financial support. There are a number of explanations for this. First, I was a proven entity within the institution. I had been with UPMC for seven years. I had run the Primary Care Internal Medicine Residency Program for five years, had acted as an ethics consultant for the hospital, and had served on many hospital committees. More important, I had done a great deal of research and writing on ethical issues associated with organ donation. Many of these projects had overlapped with the work of the Department of Surgery when Dr. Simmons had been its chair. Moreover, Dr. Simmons had conducted research on organ donation and thus had particular interest in that work. His late wife, an internationally known sociologist, had studied living-related organ donation. Dr. Simmons knew of my abilities and trusted my judgment.

Second, I had personal ties to Dr. Simmons. His significant other was a member of the Division of General Internal Medicine. Her research interest was concerned with medical ethics and the history of medicine, and I had worked closely with her during the previous five years in the Center for Bioethics and Health Law. We had worked together on a multitude of educational programs in medical ethics. Third, in an effort to convince Dr. Simmons of the worthiness of a new palliative care service, I flew to Chicago, where he was attending the American College of Surgery meeting. With the help of Dr. Charles von Gunten, we organized a visit to Northwestern's Palliative Care Service. We walked Dr. Simmons through the unit, went over its yearly patient care numbers, and reviewed its budget projections. He was quite

impressed by the high level of patient care the program provided.

The program appealed to Dr. Simmons for professional, personal, and pragmatic reasons. He understood the limitations of end-of-life care in large academic institutions because of his work as a renal transplant surgeon and because his wife had died two years earlier of metastatic breast cancer. Our arguments regarding the lack of bereavement services for families after the patients' deaths were especially persuasive to him. Pragmatically speaking, the data from our needs assessment and from the National Hospice Study convinced him that a palliative care consultation service could save money by shortening patients' hospital stays.

The program also appealed to him because it carried little risk. The Project on Death in America allowed me to spend a considerable amount of my time developing the program, time that would otherwise have required institutional funds. Dr. Simmons had to fund only the full-time nurse, the half of a physician FTE (full-time equivalent) for performing consults (minus the amount we brought in through billing), and a half-time secretary. The program therefore cost much less than the previous proposal for a 12-bed hospice unit.

With Dr. Simmons' support, we were able to move rapidly. Funding was promised less than three months after discussions began. We were able to hire a nurse practitioner through the case management program, administered by Lisa Painter and Lyda Dye, that Dr. Simmons directed. Administrative support was provided by both the Division of General Internal Medicine and the Institute for Performance Improvement, under its executive director, April Langford. We were able to start conducting consultations less than six months after our first committee meeting, a very brief time in an institution as large as the UPMC Health System. The program started in April 1998.

 Program Development and Structure
....

Institutional Background
In 1996, approximately 1000 patients died at UPMC-Presbyterian—3.5 percent of all admissions. The patients' average age was 63.6 years. Common diagnoses included cancer (13 percent), neurological illnesses (13 percent), respiratory failure (10 percent), cirrhosis (8 percent), infectious illness (6 percent), and coronary artery disease (5 percent). More than 60 percent of those who died had been in an ICU at some time during their final illness, and more than 50 percent died in the ICU. Patients who die in the hospital are "high resource utilizers." They stay significantly longer than those who are discharged alive (12.23 days vs. 6.29 days).

Average daily charges for patients who die are almost twice the charges for those who survive discharge ($9,901 vs. $5,363). UPMC-Presbyterian is a tertiary care hospital; it is probably the leading transplant center in the United States, and it has renowned oncology, neurosurgery, and cardiovascular programs.

UPMC-Shadyside, an affiliate, is a community hospital. Approximately 700 patients die there each year. Their average stay is 9.5 days. The average daily charges are lower than at UPMC-Presbyterian. Just under 50 percent of the deaths at UPMC-Shadyside occur in the ICU. A high proportion of patients die of cardiovascular disease (42 percent); others die of infection (20 percent), neurological causes (10 percent), cancer (10 percent), and pulmonary disease (10 percent). This hospital has a lower acuity than UPMC-Presbyterian. (This may be changing: the Cancer Institute and all inpatient cancer care has recently moved to Shadyside.)

UPMC-Presbyterian and UPMC-Shadyside had an interesting political relationship when the Palliative Care Service began. At the time, the two hospitals were merging. Each institution felt great stress and feared that its level of support would be diminished. The UPMC administration saw the Palliative Care Service as a program that could link the two institutions by promoting quality care at the end of life.

Staffing and Program Development

A nurse conducts the daily activities of the Service. We wanted to hire a nurse practitioner or an advanced practice nurse with specific expertise in palliative care. After an extensive search, we hired a nurse practitioner who had previously worked in an oncology unit and at a local hospice.

His hiring was the most important and most successful decision the program made in its first year. The nurse practitioner possessed excellent communication skills, knowledge of various hospices in Pittsburgh, and the emotional ability to handle crises and deaths with equanimity. A new service must be able to sell itself to many different constituencies. This nurse practitioner is highly engaging and personable. He made friends with nurses, doctors, and social workers throughout the institution, and he dealt with critically ill patients with warmth and sensitivity. Because our initial role was largely to provide emotional support and negotiate with patients and their families regarding treatment goals, his strengths were ideally suited to the Service. His previous experience in hospice meant that he knew, better than anyone else on the team, what community resources were available. The pressure to shorten hospital stays and the emotional tenor of many of our consultations made the nurse practitioner's job very stressful. His ability to stay calm and good-humored, amid what often seemed chaotic, was amazing.

The other paid staff person is a physician. Three physicians originally worked on the Service: a geriatrician, an oncologist, and me—a general internist. Given our primary specialties, we were all familiar with the care of terminally ill patients. The two other doctors had also served as the medical co-directors of hospice—experience that did not prepare them for our consult service.

A doctor of pharmacy serves as a consultant to the Service. Luckily, the pharmacist who manages the UPCI pain service volunteered for this role. Colleagues widely view her as UPMC's most knowledgeable person regarding pain therapy. None of the physicians had extensive training in pain management. Particularly in the early days of our program, she acted as the pain expert, advised us about cases, and educated us about therapeutics. Having been at UPCI for more than 10 years, she is also a useful connection to the oncology service.

A psychologist agreed to provide in-depth psychosocial counseling and assessment, case by case. The UPMC Cancer Institute Behavioral Medicine Service provided a postdoctoral student with experience in consultations, at no cost. The addition of this participant allowed us to provide psychological care for patients and their families. Moreover, she serves as the psychological back-up for the volunteers who work on the bereavement service. She attends all weekly multidisciplinary meetings and provides feedback and guidance on psychological issues for the rest of the team.

The director of the Chaplaincy service and a social worker from the oncology service act as consultants to the team. A volunteer coordinator and two volunteers provide bereavement and follow-up services.

Finally, a secretary receives and directs requests for consultations, helps collect data, distributes sympathy cards, and performs other administrative tasks.

Administrative Structure

The Palliative Care Service has a complex administrative structure because it is funded by the Institute for Performance Improvement but is conducted through the Division of General Internal Medicine. For example, the nurse practitioner reports to the director of Case Management, who has specific ideas about how he should relate to case managers and social workers. Yet, the nurse practitioner spends much of his clinical time working with the palliative care physicians. As the director of the Palliative Care Service, I therefore supervise most of his daily responsibilities. This led to

confusion that required careful discussion between the director of Case Management and me. (As of March 2000, the nurse practitioners began reporting directly to the Section of Palliative Care and Medical Ethics.) The institute pays part of my salary and I serve as its associate director in charge of Palliative Care and Family Support; because I report directly to Dr. Simmons in that capacity, I have experienced little role conflict. My responsibilities to the Institute and to the Division of General Internal Medicine harmonize; both require me to build a palliative care program. We accomplish much of the daily work and administration of the Palliative Care Service within the Division of General Internal Medicine. The same division houses the Section of Palliative Care and Medical Ethics and the Section is responsible to that division.

UPCI and the Institute of Performance Improvement assign the social workers to work with us on administrative and psychosocial support for critically ill patients; the pharmacist, clergy, and volunteers donated their time. Our psychologist initially volunteered but now bills for her consultations. We have tried to deal with such administrative complications by developing a Steering Committee at UPMC-Shadyside and UPMC-Presbyterian. We do not know if the Steering Committee will allow us to more efficiently plan our clinical time.

Another complication is that the UPMC Hospice has a completely separate administrative structure. Moreover, a different corporation runs the hospice. Attempts have been made to combine the two services into one palliative care service; however, the administrative distance between the two programs has made these efforts unsuccessful. (In February 2000, talks were resumed to see if the two programs could be better integrated.)

Program Operations

Consultations are available seven days a week, 24 hours a day. Attending physicians—or house staff, with the attending physician's permission—can request a consultation. All consultation requests are directed to a central phone number. During weekday working hours, this number reaches the palliative care secretary; at other times, the caller reaches an answering service. The secretary or answering service notifies the palliative care attending or nurse practitioner of the request. Within two hours, the patient's attending physician or the house staff is contacted and asked about the consultation's goals. The consultative service reviews all pathology and radiology studies, interviews and examines the patient, and meets with the family before making formal recommendations. To facilitate our evaluation, we developed a structured intake form. It combines questions from the

Edmonton System Assessment Scale, the McGill Quality of Life Scale; and the Missoula-VITAS Quality of Life Scale: assessments of activities of daily living (ADLs); and questions regarding the patient's cognitive ability. With input from the social workers, nutritionists, and chaplains, we added questions about nutritional, spiritual, and financial matters. We also included questions about patients' understanding of their disease and prognosis, their interest in discussing living wills, and the identity of their surrogate decision makers. (Our initial attempts to develop a structured intake form were unsuccessful. Most staffers found it long and cumbersome, and it was filled out less than 10 percent of the time. We recently shortened the form and, with a renewed commitment, will try to fill it out for each patient.)

We also developed a form for families. It is meant to find out the family's views of their loved one's illness and prognosis; to understand their medical, psychosocial, spiritual, and financial concerns; and to assess their support systems. Our goal is to meet with the family within 24 hours of the consultation. In more than 95 percent of the cases, we have met that goal.

Consultations are completed within 24 hours. After the palliative care attending and nurse practitioner have seen the patient and assessed the case, referrals are made to other members of the team:

- a palliative care psychologist, to help the patient or family with psychological issues;
- a doctor of pharmacy with expertise in pain management, who reviews the chart and recommends therapy;
- a wound care nurse, who makes recommendations for skin care;
- a spiritual counselor for the patient and family; and
- the primary social worker who is assigned to the patient, for patient and family support and for help with discharge planning if it is appropriate.

To date, we have not worked with the ethics consultation service. Because members of the palliative care team also serve as ethics consultants, they have not needed formal ethics consultations.

Initially, we expected that most of our consults would be for symptom management. During the first year, communication with the patient and family regarding psychosocial issues, advance directives, and disposition turned out to be more common reasons for consultation. However, once we performed a formal evaluation, we often found that symptoms were adversely affecting the quality of life. Control of these symptoms not only enhances that quality but also lets patients communicate openly with their families about their goals and plan for end-of-life care.

We also spend a great deal of time providing support to families. The nurse practitioner and the primary social worker meet with families every day to provide psychosocial support and to help with financial issues and discharge planning. Our behavioral medicine psychologist meets with families who have been identified as having special needs. She discusses ways to improve the patient's quality of life simply, such as by wearing a perfume that the patient likes, playing the patient's favorite music, or watching familiar television shows with her or him. The behavioral medicine psychologist also explains how the family can cope with their loved one's serious illness.

The palliative care attending calls the referring physician with our recommendations. The nurse practitioner coordinates the plan of care with behavioral medicine, social work, nutritional, and pastoral care to ensure that the needs in each of those areas are met. The nurse practitioner and pharmacist educate the patient and family, as well as the nursing staff and auxiliary personnel, about the plan of care; to coordinate counseling with the social worker; and work with the case managers on discharge planning. We follow patients daily until their discharge. Then the service calls the hospice caring for the patient at home, home care provider, or nursing home to which the patient is being discharged and discusses the plan of care. If we discharge the patient to a nursing home, we contact the facility again one week after discharge to follow up and to help solve problems with the primary team (the doctors and nurses who have a long-term relationship with the patient).

Once a week, we discuss all patients (generally between 3 and 10) in a multidisciplinary meeting, which includes the doctor of pharmacy, social workers, psychologists, bereavement counselor, spiritual counselors, physician, and nurse practitioner. Team members present the cases of all patients seen during the week, and the team discusses how to improve their care.

Follow Up and Bereavement
Grief and bereavement services are a major part of the Palliative Care Service. We provide four programs: a follow-up program for patients who are still alive, a bereavement program for families of patients who have died in the hospital, a family support program for families of critically ill patients newly admitted to the ICU, and a program for health care providers.

Patients who are discharged continue to need palliative care. Patients were frequently being readmitted only one or two weeks after discharge for management of pain or other symptoms. In talking with their families, we learned that the lack of continuity between intensive, hospital-based palliative care and home or nursing home care was a problem. Inadequate communication between the primary hospital service and the nursing home or home care provider caused confusion and misinterpretation. That is why we developed a follow-up program for all palliative care patients who are discharged.

We call both the physician who will care for the patient at home and the home nursing provider to supply information about the patient's and family's understanding of the illness and prognosis, about symptom-based treatments, and about psychosocial and spiritual issues. If we discharge the patient to a nursing home, we also call one week after discharge to help ensure adequate care and to answer any questions the patient or caregivers may have. If there are clinical questions, we talk to the primary physician to ensure that the patient and family are given consistent messages.

We trained a volunteer to make monthly follow-up calls to patients. These calls serve two purposes. First, we want patients to know that we care about them and want them to continue to receive the best palliative care possible. (If clinical issues arise, the volunteer calls the clinical service, which then talks with the primary health care providers.) Second, we want to know when the patient dies, so we can enroll the family in our bereavement program.

Few U.S. hospitals have a coordinated bereavement program for families of patients who die. The first thing—and often the only thing—that a family receives after their loved one dies is a hospital bill. We thought we could do better than that. Therefore, we developed a comprehensive bereavement program for the families of all patients for whom we had consulted. Families can enroll in the bereavement program in one of two ways. Families of all patients who die in the hospital are automatically entered in the program. If our follow-up phone calls reveal that a non-hospice patient has died, we enter the family in the program. (We exclude patients at hospices. They have bereavement programs of their own, and we do not want to duplicate services.)

As part of the bereavement program, we ask the doctors and nurses on the unit on which the patient died to sign a sympathy card, which we mail to the patient's family. Later we send the family a monthly newsletter developed by the National Hospice Organization and mailed by volunteers at the UPMC Hospice. Then we have a trained volunteer follow up. She calls each family one month, three months, six months, and 12 months after the death to see how the family is doing. Our psychologist has supplied her with a list of community resources and serves as a consultant for difficult situations.

In the first year of service we performed consults for 324 patients; 93 of them died in the hospital. All of their families are being followed by the bereavement program. Of the remaining 231 patients, who were discharged to hospice, to a nursing facility, or to a private home, 105 have died. We are following their families, except for those who receive bereavement services through hospice.

These three programs provide psychosocial support to grieving patients and families. However, health care providers also grieve. During our consultations, we found that doctors and nurses often have strong emotional responses to their patients' deaths. When a unit has a series of difficult deaths, staff comment on how it affects their lives and ability to care for other patients. We therefore formed a team consisting of the head chaplain, the palliative care nurse practitioner, and an oncology social worker to provide psychosocial support for health care providers who are grieving over patient loss. In addition to allowing the staff to talk about their feelings, the team also teaches coping mechanisms and provides referrals if staff members want additional counseling.

To publicize the bereavement program for staff members, we used meetings with each nurse manager, informal communications, and flyers on each unit. We have conducted approximately ten grief sessions for health care providers. A representative case involved the death of a young woman injured in a motor vehicle accident. She was pregnant at the time, subsequently aborted a stillborn baby in the ICU, and then died herself. The nurses on the unit had experience with the death of young adults but were having a very difficult time dealing with the stillbirth. A bereavement session allowed the nurses to vent their feelings about the tragic event. Staff were also able to discuss how their feelings influenced their personal lives and to learn about techniques that could help them deal with those feelings.

Publicity and Public Relations
Because the Palliative Care Service began at UPMC-Presbyterian, we began to publicize it there. We held meetings in every division within the Department of Medicine as well as with most major programs in the Department of Surgery. I met individually with the top 10 admitters to the hospital and with each critical-care medicine and pulmonary doctor who works in the intensive care unit. The nurse practitioner and physicians developed a 15-minute talk on palliative care and the Service's goals and mission. I also called some of the attending physicians for whom we had done consults to ask for feedback and find out how we could better meet their needs. We also prepared a

brochure to introduce the program to physicians and to patients and their families.

We developed an intensive outreach program with the house staff. We went to morning report at least twice a week to inquire about patients and visited the ICU daily. When performing consults, we asked the house staff to join us so we could show them how to communicate regarding sensitive issues. We also used our notes as an opportunity to educate the house staff. In addition, we developed formal educational programs on palliative care for the internal medicine residents, the geriatrics and oncology fellows, and the critical medicine program. For good measure, we provided chocolates and other refreshments to the house staff.

We prepared a similar outreach program for other health care providers at UPMC-Presbyterian. The nurse practitioner conducted in-service sessions on every unit and every intensive care unit within six months after the program started. We met with nurse practitioners, social workers, case managers, and chaplains. The nurse practitioner made rounds with the oncology nurses and went to their multidisciplinary meetings to learn about patients who are most appropriate for palliative care consults.

We developed an outreach and publicity program at UPMC-Shadyside as well. The general hospital newsletter and the physicians' newsletter published articles about the Comprehensive Palliative Care Service. I met with the hospital auxiliary committee, which promised to support our bereavement program. The Shadyside Foundation agreed to send out fundraising letters to the community.

We also tried to meet with many members of the house staff and attending physicians at UPMC-Shadyside to increase our visibility and encourage requests for consultations. I met with the head of the Department of Medicine and of the Department of Surgery and attended meetings of division chiefs in both departments. We also met with the doctors who ran the intensive care units and with the highest admitters on the medical and surgical services. I began participating in morning report on the medical service and conducted conferences on palliative care for the internal medicine and family medicine residents. The nurse practitioner conducted a number of inservice sessions and attended multidisciplinary meetings on the oncology floor.

We met with public relations staff responsible for internal and external publicity at UPMC Health System. Press releases regarding the program have run in the UPMC newsletter and the physicians' newsletter. UPMC sponsored ads in local newspapers. Articles about the program have

appeared in the University of Pittsburgh magazine and the University of Pittsburgh Medical School magazine. Both of the city's newspapers, local health-related television and radio programs, and the national media have covered the Service.

Program Growth

The program has expanded three times. Initially, we saw patients only at UPMC-Presbyterian. Although the two hospitals are less than three miles apart, we wanted to be sure that our policies and procedures worked and that we could provide good service in one setting before expanding. In October 1998, we expanded our consult service to UPMC-Shadyside. This coincided with the move to that hospital of the University of Pittsburgh Cancer Institute, which had requested many of our consults. The UPMC-Shadyside administration agreed to fund a half-time nurse practitioner so that we would be more visible to the hospital's residents.

Despite our vigorous efforts to publicize the program, we have been less successful in obtaining consultations at UPMC-Shadyside than at UPMC-Presbyterian. The environment of Shadyside is that of a private hospital. Consults are organized and directed by the private attending physicians, with little input from the house staff. Physicians' referral patterns are ingrained, and it is quite difficult for "outsiders" to become involved.

Moreover, a measure of ill will arose during the merger between UPMC-Shadyside and UPMC-Presbyterian. Shadyside saw us as a UPMC-Presbyterian service, as outside academicians who were being brought in to tell the private doctors how to practice palliative care. This was not a helpful perception. In fact, Shadyside greeted the nurse practitioner with a fair amount of anger and distrust. Despite this, the number of consults increased monthly during her work at UPMC-Shadyside. Unfortunately, she left at the end of four months because she felt unwelcome and because of the stress of caring for terminally ill hospitalized patients; owing to budget issues, we have not hired someone to fill this position. The lack of a consistent health care provider presence at UPMC-Shadyside has interfered with our ability to build up the Service.

Family Support and Organ Donation
In March 1999 at UPMC-Presbyterian, problems with organ donation presented another opportunity to improve the care of the families of critically ill patients. Under the current nationwide organ allocation rules, local organ-procurement rates obviously have a large impact on an institution's supply of organs for transplantation. The UPMC Health System has one of the busiest and best known transplant programs in the United States.

The lack of donated organs prevents still more transplants from being performed. UPMC-Presbyterian's overall consent rate was 47 percent—about the national average—but it ranged from 30 to 65 percent in different areas of the hospital. Because of my previous research in this area and my involvement in the Institute for Performance Improvement, I was asked to develop interventions that would improve consent rates for organ donation.

Data suggest that families whose loved ones have a potentially life-threatening illness lack support and information. In the course of conducting palliative care consultations, we were struck by the "culture shock" that families experience when a loved one is admitted to an ICU. In addition to the emotions evoked by the illness itself, families are not prepared for the ICU's environment or structure. We were involved in a number of cases in which families reacted negatively, causing a great deal of distress in the ICU. Families under stress may also be less likely to donate organs and may regret that choice later on. To rectify this problem, ICU nurses, social workers, and members of our local organ-procurement program worked with us to develop a family support program. This program is designed to provide psychosocial and spiritual help to families whose loved ones are likely to die. Eventually, we want to extend this program to every family whose loved one is admitted to the ICU. The program has the following components:

- The social worker or nurse caring for the patient identifies the patient as being at high risk of dying. Criteria for high risk include having a Glasgow Coma Scale of 6 or less; having a DNR order; receiving comfort care only; having decided to forgo life-sustaining treatment; or having a subjective judgment that the patient will die during the next three days.

- The family support contact person, that is, a social worker trained in palliative care, the palliative care nurse practitioner, or the palliative care attending physician, talks with the people who are caring for the patient about how the family is coping. The contact person asks about spiritual help, financial needs, psychosocial concerns, and family dynamics.

- The primary nurse assesses the family's understanding of the patient's condition, and identifies family sources of support. The nurse offers psychosocial support and offers to contact a spiritual counselor. The nurse or social worker also provides basic information that the family will need, such as the locations of hospital restrooms and showers, and local restaurants, pharmacies, and places of worship. We give the family a pamphlet describing the ICU's structure and visiting hours, and we provide a list of important names and phone numbers (i.e., the unit's number and the names of the ICU doctors and primary nurse).

- We document information on a family support flow chart and place it in the medical record so that other health care providers understand how the family is doing.

- The social worker works with the primary team to schedule daily meetings to bring the family up to date regarding the patient's prognosis and current medical treatment.

- We also developed two assessment forms. The first is used every day to assess the family's needs and to provide feedback to the health care team regarding what can be done to help the family. We send the second form to families after discharge and use it to assess the efficacy of the entire family support program.

- We automatically enter families of patients who die in the ICU into the bereavement program.

To staff this program, the Institute for Performance Improvement agreed to pay half of a physician FTE and to hire three extra social workers for evening and nighttime shifts.

In the spring of 1998, we began the family support program in the neurosurgical ICU. Feedback from the staff has been very positive. They report that the program has improved relations with families. Informal feedback from families has also been positive. Formal program evaluation is scheduled to start in the fall of 2000. We want to modify this program to meet the needs of other intensive care units.

ICU Patients and Palliative Care

We developed a program to identify ICU patients who need palliative care referrals. ICU nurses enter the APACHE scores of all patients admitted to the ICU in a computer database; patients whose score is associated with a 75 percent mortality upon admission, a 50 percent mortality on the fifth hospital day, or any score on the fourteenth hospital day are considered possible palliative care candidates. Twice a week, we speak with the primary nurse care coordinator about these patients. Doing so lets us develop a better relationship with the head nurses in the ICU. Despite these patients' high risk of dying, few doctors had discussed end-of-life issues with the patient or family. This led us to revise our educational program for ICU physicians and to work with units on developing guidelines for physician-family conferences. The critical care physicians who helped develop this project presented it

as an abstract for the 1999 national meeting of the American College of Chest Physicians.

This program has allowed us to collaborate with people in the Division of Critical Care Medicine. Two physicians are working with us on research projects involving both critical care and palliative care, while a Ph.D. researcher has developed an intervention for families of critically ill patients. Another physician has joined the program as a consultant.

Developing Institutional Ties

We have worked hard to maintain good lines of communication within the UPMC Health Care System. To maintain political and economic support, I have written monthly memoranda to Dr. Simmons, Dr. Kapoor, Dr. Trump (head of UPCI), Joyce Yasko (associate director of UPCI Clinical Programs and Network), and many other policymakers within the institution. These memos report the number of patients for whom we have performed consults; describe one or two patients whom we affected significantly, either by increasing psychosocial care or decreasing health care costs; and describe our educational and research accomplishments.

I meet quarterly with the leaders of UPMC-Presbyterian and UPMC-Shadyside. These meetings with the hospitals' chief executive officers, chief financial officers, and boards allow me to bring them up to date regarding our successes, obtain their input regarding areas in which we are having trouble, and review new proposals and initiatives.

We developed three other outreach programs to try to ensure our clinical success. First, all of the palliative care physicians joined the UPCI faculty, which helped reassure the oncologists that I was part of their team. Second, when issues arise or health care providers report problems with our Service, we respond promptly and work very hard to resolve these issues. If we do not provide excellent service to the primary team, we view it as an emergency that must be rectified. Third, we have worked closely with the house staff. Initially, we publicized our Service through gifts of chocolate and daily reminders at morning report and during rounds. This helped bring us wide visibility with the medicine and surgical house staff. We continually give presentations about palliative care to medical services within the institution. While we have received only a few consults from services such as physical medicine and rehabilitation or general psychiatry, they have often recommended that other services request a consultation.

In addition to providing educational services and trying to influence formal mechanisms of power and referral within the institution, we have used informal routes to maintain visibility. The nurse practitioner and I have given talks at Family House, a place where families stay at very low cost when their loved ones are in the hospital, as well as to the auxiliary clubs at UPMC-Shadyside and UPMC-Presbyterian. We have presented talks to a number of board and staff committees, hoping to educate them regarding palliative care in general and the staff and function of the Service in particular.

We act as a resource for other institutions that wish to build palliative care consulting services. We have sent information about our program, including our business plan and intake forms, to more than ten university programs and three community hospitals. We spoke with the staffs at a number of these programs by phone, answering questions about our program. Representatives of a hospice in Erie, Pennsylvania, and West Virginia University Hospital each visited us for a day to obtain more information.

Program Status
· ·

Core Program: Results of the First Year
In the first year, the Palliative Care Service was consulted in 347 cases. They constituted 14 percent of all ICU deaths at UPMC-Presbyterian and 27 percent of non-ICU

deaths. Like palliative care services elsewhere, we found that most patients for whom we consulted had end-stage cancer (73 percent). The Service has followed patients with various types of cancer including: lung (15 percent), hematological (14 percent), GI (14 percent), liver (10 percent), and breast (8 percent). Other diseases included neurological conditions such as stroke and subarachnoid hemorrhage (7 percent), end-stage heart failure (5 percent), chronic obstructive lung disease (5 percent), cirrhosis (4 percent), renal failure (1 percent), AIDS (1 percent), and various other diagnoses (4 percent). Since the family support program began, we have been involved with a larger number of brain hemorrhages, motor vehicle accidents, and other acute neurological events.

We have obtained consultations from every unit in the hospital. They include: general medicine floors (57 percent—22 percent of which were on the oncology floors), ICUs (24 percent), surgical units (16 percent), and outpatient, emergency room, and rehabilitation units (3 percent).

Patients' ages ranged from 22 to 97, with an average age of 64 years. Fifty-one percent of the patients were male and 49 percent were white. Their religious affiliations were Catholic (49 percent), Protestant (21 percent), Jewish (5 percent), and other faiths (25 percent). Most patients

had Medicare insurance (53 percent); a smaller percentage had Medicaid or private insurance (46 percent), and a few were self-insured (1 percent).

Patients stayed in the hospital an average of 12.2 days before the Palliative Care Service became involved. (The number of days ranged from 1 to 130.) We completed 95 percent of consultations within one day of the request. The reasons we were consulted included: communication regarding end-of-life, family support, and discharge planning (95 percent) and symptom management, such as pain, nausea and vomiting, shortness of breath, constipation, anorexia and cachexia, and depression and anxiety (25 percent). (Percentages exceed 100 percent because there was more than one reason for some consultations.) Although consults were requested for symptom management in only 25 percent of cases, we identified and made suggestions regarding physical symptoms in 95 percent of cases.

The palliative care psychologist met with 93 patients and families during the first year. She followed many patients at home with UPMC Hospice via phone calls and interactions with the hospice nurses.

Of the patients for whom we performed consults, approximately 33 percent died in the hospital. Another 25 percent were sent to a nursing home, and 40 percent went home. More than three quarters of those who went home went with a home hospice consultation. Most of the others were followed by a home health nursing service that was oriented toward palliative care. Approximately 30 other patients were discharged directly to an inpatient hospice.

The Palliative Care Service started at Shadyside Hospital in October 1998. Since then we performed consults for 41 patients. The initial reasons for consults were family support (85 percent), symptom management (43 percent), and discharge planning (10 percent). Of the 41 patients, 26 percent died in the hospital; the rest were discharged to hospice (37 percent), nursing facilities (23 percent), or home (14 percent). The ages of the patients ranged from 18 to 96, with an average age of 59 years. Their religious affiliations were: Catholic (45 percent), Protestant (29 percent), and others (26 percent). The majority of the patients were female (61 percent).

Of the 324 patients for whom we performed consults at either hospital, 198 died within our first year. All of these families were enrolled in our bereavement program. We also included families of 38 patients who died at home and who were not in a hospice program.

Program Evaluation
At UPMC-Presbyterian we sent evaluation forms to the attending physician, the house staff, the primary nurse, and the patient or family. In the first six weeks, we received 60 responses—17 from patients' families and 43 from health care providers. These evaluations were extraordinarily positive. More than 88 percent of the families reported that they were satisfied or very satisfied with the availability of our team and satisfied or very satisfied with the way the team included the family in decisions about treatment and care. They appreciated the opportunities to talk with members of the palliative care team.

Unfortunately, as the number of consults increased, it was not practical to ask health care providers to fill out a two-page evaluation form after every consult, particularly on units where we performed up to two consultations per week. Moreover, we had difficulty getting attendings and families to return the evaluation form. We therefore stopped requesting evaluations after every consultation.

Health Care Provider Evaluation
After six months of the consultation service, we sent surveys to internal medicine residents, all primary nurse care coordinators (PNCCs), and all social workers and case managers. Sixty surveys were returned by the internal medicine house staff, 24 by the PNCCs, and 21 by the social workers.

Of the 60 physicians, 36 had participated in at least one palliative care consult during the study period. These physicians reported high levels of satisfaction with the Palliative Care Service. Ninety-seven percent of the respondents were satisfied or very satisfied with the Service's recommendations. One hundred percent thought our recommendations were timely and addressed the medical and psychosocial issues. Ninety-four percent of the physicians thought the Service helped them deal with families, and 89 percent believed the consult improved patient care. Eighty-three percent reported that the Service taught them something about palliative care. Ninety-seven percent of respondents reported that they would use the Service again.

The PNCC survey results were also very positive. Of the 22 respondents who had participated in consults, 91 percent were satisfied or very satisfied with the Service's recommendations. Ninety-five percent thought the recommendations were timely and addressed the medical and psychosocial issues. Eighty-six percent of respondents thought the Service helped them deal with families, and 82 percent believed the consult improved patient care. Eighty-six percent reported that the Service taught them something about palliative care. Ninety-one percent reported that they would use the Service again.

No formal evaluations of the Service have been completed at UPMC-Shadyside. We have recently developed an evaluation form for the family support program. This form will be tested in three units—the neurological intensive care unit, the cardiology care unit, and the medical ICU.

Here is one example of how we helped a family to choose care that was appropriate for the patient and family:

We saw a 73-year-old woman with end-stage breast cancer and acute renal failure. The patient was minimally responsive and unable to make decisions about her medical care. Hospital personnel had not approached her about advance directives. The family had been having a very difficult time with the patient's terminal state and with her poor quality of life during several previous weeks. We met with the family and asked whether, when she was alert and oriented, they had ever discussed what the patient would want if she became this ill. The family said that they had indeed discussed the matter and that the patient had said she never wanted to have her life prolonged in this way. We established goals with the family and concentrated upon her comfort. We recommended that her lab work and IVs be stopped and her NG tube removed. We sought to relieve her pain, dyspnea (death rattle), and agitation. The patient was transferred to a local inpatient hospice the following day and died a short time later.

When we called the family as part of our bereavement program, they noted that they were very pleased with her care.

Fiscal Implications

Physician services are billed as consultations. It has been hard to determine our billable income because there were large differences in billing by different physicians. We are working with the billing department to develop consistent standards. That department has agreed to review our notes and billing every three months and advise us regarding our practices. The department is also trying to untangle some of the more complicated billing rules. For example, we were initially told that if the primary physician is a general internist, another general internist could not bill for a consult. Later we were told that we would be reimbursed in these situations after all, but further investigation is needed. The question is whether both internists are billing for the same diagnosis. Because we focus on symptoms rather than diagnoses, we are working with the billing office to develop billing cards that are symptom- as well as diagnosis-based. The cards will emphasize billing for counseling, which is a large part of what we do. The office is giving us quarterly reports of our billing and collections so that we can assess the impact of the changes that have already been made.

We have begun to raise money from charitable sources. In our first year, approximately $15,000 was raised through an appeal at UPMC-Shadyside. We raised another $8,000 from drug companies to support our educational efforts. Finally, the auxiliary committees from the two hospitals have contributed approximately $1,000, which we used to subsidize our bereavement program.

These revenues do not take into account the money the Palliative Care Service saved. Based on the National Hospice Study, we predicted that we would reduce ancillary care costs by 40 percent and shorten hospital stays by one day per patient. It is impossible to assess these savings without a randomized trial using a control group. However, our monthly reports try to document cases in which we believe savings have occurred. Such savings are very important; clinical billings are unlikely to raise enough money to support the Service.

In addition to these attempts to raise money, members of the Service have submitted numerous grant proposals in 1998–1999. The grant from the Project on Death in America gave me the time to begin the program. Subsequently, Susan Block and I received a grant from the Nathan Cummings Foundation that has allowed me to fund 50 percent of the psychologist on the Palliative Care Service to study how doctors respond to their patients' deaths. During 1999, faculty from the Service submitted seven grant proposals to the NIH and to private foundations.

In the long run, research funding is vital to the Palliative Care Service's survival for two reasons. In an academic environment, research provides intellectual cachet. Research grants show the rest of the university that the Service is a scholarly endeavor. As important, we can use our research funds to improve our clinical mission by increasing our knowledge base and allowing us to stretch our resources where clinical and research activities overlap. By collecting data that would otherwise be unobtainable, research can improve our clinical work, as well as our base of knowledge. For example, we have been unable to free staff members to obtain patient or family satisfaction data after our interventions. We found it difficult to have a staff person available to meet with the family before a patient was discharged to ensure completion of the evaluation forms. However, Ellen Redinbaugh, the Service's psychologist, received an NIH grant to study a psychoeducational intervention on caregivers of terminally ill hospice patients. She is attempting to enroll patients from the Palliative Care Service for this study. As part

of this process, she has volunteered to have her staff meet with patients before their discharge, to obtain our satisfaction data and to talk with them about her study. Thus we can collect data we could not obtain in any other fashion.

Program Obstacles

The program has faced a number of obstacles during its development and its first year. One problem was staffing. Three physicians originally shared clinical responsibilities. The oncologist, who was expected to spend three months on the Service, quit after the first month because of the time it required, although he has remained very supportive of the program within the Division of Oncology. That left only two physicians. At the end of the first year, the geriatrician decided not to continue performing consults. His previous experience was as a hospice medical director, and the shift from that role to being an inpatient palliative care physician was too great. He had philosophical difficulties providing palliative care to dying patients who wanted aggressive treatment nonetheless. Moreover, his major interest is in symptom management, and our Service's emphasis on psychosocial care tempered his enjoyment of the work. He did not like the uncertainty and stress associated with a consulting service. He decided to withdraw from palliative and hospice care and concentrate on geriatrics. This meant that I was the only physician performing clinical consultations for eight of the first 12 months of the Service. Our 24-hour-a-day, seven-day-a-week service made this much more wearing than I had anticipated. It also kept me from attending to essential administrative, educational, and research matters.

To handle this problem, we have hired two new physicians. One is a board-certified general internist with a fellowship in palliative care. The second is a general internist with a master's degree in medical ethics. He attended a three-day conference on palliative care and is engaged in an independent study using the American Academy of Hospice and Palliative Medicine's UNIPAC material and the *Oxford Textbook of Palliative Care*. Before hiring these physicians, I discussed the Service's philosophy and the time commitment it requires more explicitly than I had with the oncologist and geriatrician. Although it is important that these two physicians supplement our staff, the Service may be hurt by the lack of an oncologist.

We had a similar problem in nursing. Initially, we hired a half-time nurse practitioner to staff UPMC-Shadyside. While she had extensive experience at an inpatient hospice, she found that our work was quite different. Our work consists largely of crisis

management, and relationships with patients and families, while intense, are brief (average time from initial consult to discharge is four days; median is two). The nurse was inexperienced in trying to combine palliative care and aggressive life-prolonging measures. After six months, she resigned.

We are also too dependent on the kindness of other programs for our non-physician staff. Currently, the only dedicated staff members employed in the Palliative Care Service are the full-time nurse practitioner and the three physicians (paid .5 FTE for their time on the consultative service). Other staff—the psychologist, chaplain, social worker, and pharmacist—are all volunteers. Thus their primary allegiance is not always to the Palliative Care Service. When schedules are tight and they are needed elsewhere, they are unable to devote as much time to palliative care. This interferes with our ability to have a multidisciplinary team, provide comprehensive end-of-life care to patients, and educate the staff throughout UPMC.

We have no dedicated administrator, either. We have patched together administrative support from various sources, and these personnel have done an admirable job. However, the lack of a dedicated administrator limits our ability to think strategically about how to improve the Service and make it financially viable. For example, we now do very little to evaluate our impact on patient care. This will become increasingly important if we are to justify our existence. A dedicated administrator could identify possible funding sources, raise money, monitor the financial strength of the service as it grows, manage grants, work on development efforts, and analyze billing for clinical services.

An unexpected problem during our first year involved our poor relationship with social workers at UPMC-Shadyside and UPMC-Presbyterian. Social workers' roles within the UPMC Health Care System have been changing rapidly. The institution's support for a Palliative Care Service, especially one that is led by a physician and that concentrates chiefly on family counseling, may have caused conflict with social workers, whose jobs included counseling. The Service's use of a psychologist may have offended some, since this kind of consultation has also been the social workers' traditional responsibility. My explanation that we were using the psychologist because she volunteered her time did little to lessen their concern.

During the early months of the Service, we compounded these problems by not always contacting the social workers or involving them sufficiently in the consultations. For example, the nurse practitioner, who had a great deal of experience working with home hospices, often took it upon himself to arrange for follow-up with home hospices. He did not always understand patients' insurance, and the social workers thought he was promising services that they could not deliver.

We tried to solve these problems by improving communication and participation. The social workers do know the patients and families better than any other health care providers, and they also understand the complicated fiscal environment. By increasing their involvement in our consultations, we have improved patient care. They, and we, have gained a better appreciation of our respective knowledge and skills. I have also tried to correct the perception that we do not respect or care about social workers. A social worker has joined our Steering Committee, and at least one social worker now attends all of our multidisciplinary meetings.

We have had more difficulty than I anticipated obtaining requests for consults at UPMC-Shadyside. Once our part-time nurse practitioner resigned in April 1999, the number of consults gradually neared zero, although it increased slightly with the deployment of two of the palliative care physicians at Shadyside University Hospital. We have received few requests for consults from the private physicians affiliated with Shadyside, although we have repeatedly met with groups of physicians and given innumerable talks. This is discouraging despite hospital leaders' assurances that private doctors typically take two to three years to change their referral patterns. Meanwhile, the lack of consultations has led the UPMC-Shadyside administrator to reconsider the hospital's financial support. This is distressing. Without a nurse practitioner, we will have no regular presence at the hospital and will be even less apt to obtain referrals.

 Educational Endeavors

Given our limited resources, education has always been a central part of the Service. We have adopted four kinds of educational programs. First, we received a small grant from the Beckwith Foundation to train nurses on two units in the hospital to provide better palliative care. We hope to obtain referrals from these units and to turn them into palliative care satellites later.

Second, we opened the consult service to medical students, residents, fellows, and nurse practitioners. This has given students the chance to improve their clinical skills in palliative care. Two residents, one fellow, and four fourth-year medical students each spent a month with us in our first year.

Third, we have begun planning to train medical students and house staff. We have completed a yearlong needs assessment for

the medical school. More than 20 second-year medical students volunteered to help with this project by reading all course materials, reviewing the patient-based learning cases, and surveying fourth-year students and recent graduates. We have presented plans for an integrated four-year curriculum to the curriculum committee. We also have submitted an internal grant proposal for a new first-year course on hospice and palliative care. (There is a great demand for this course among students themselves. All first-year students have volunteered to make rounds with us every Saturday and Sunday. By Spring 2000, we had students signed up for rounds until the spring of 2001.) Simultaneously, we have developed curricula in communication skills for all internal medicine house staff. All members of the house staff receive a four-hour program on giving bad news to patients and families, discussing goals of therapy, and existential issues in palliative care. In addition, we have developed a model palliative care curriculum for the primary care internal medicine house staff. This curriculum consists of ten hours of discussion regarding pain and symptom management, hospice care, spiritual issues in palliative care, and grief and bereavement. Primary care house staff also attend four sessions about communicating with the critically ill, covering topics such as giving bad news, advance care planning, existential issues, and running a family meeting. Residents also spend five half-days making rounds on the inpatient palliative care service and the outpatient hospice.

Fourth, we have helped develop educational materials for many other residency training programs inside and outside of the UPMC Health Care System. We developed a curriculum for oncology and geriatric fellows and for the neurosurgery house staff. These programs, which consist of four to six sessions, cover symptom management, giving bad news, and grief and bereavement. The feedback has been quite good, and we will try to expand these sessions to other services. We also completed a series of faculty development workshops for the St. Margaret Family Residency Program. In addition, the Service has developed "grief rounds" for nurses and other health care providers. These one-hour sessions are held on units within one or two days after they are requested. The sessions help the staff examine their feelings of bereavement after patients' deaths or other losses. Approximately ten such sessions have occurred.

 Looking Forward
. . . .

In July 1999, we established a multidisciplinary palliative care clinic for outpatients. It provides pain and symptom management and follow-up care for both patients who recently left the hospital and ambulatory patientswho are referred to us. The clinic is available for patients who are not in hospices and serves as a resource for local hospice programs. The clinic is staffed by the director of the UPMC Hospice, Dr. Linda King, the palliative care nurse practitioner, a social worker, and the pharmacist from the University of Pittsburgh Cancer Institute. The outpatient office is located at Falk Clinic, which is contiguous with UPMC-Presbyterian. (When our cancer service moves into new offices in 2001, we plan to move with them.)

A second focus over the next year is how to improve our relationship with community hospices. During our first year we developed close ties to the UPMC Hospice. Established in 1997, the hospice is nonprofit, Medicare-certified, accredited by the Joint Commission on Accreditation of Healthcare Organizations (JCAHO), and licensed by the Commonwealth of Pennsylvania. In its first two years, it provided hospice and palliative care services for more than 400 patients. A large percentage of the Service's patients are discharged to the UPMC Hospice. In the first year, we referred 152 patients to its home hospice–palliative care program. Using it for our referrals markedly increases patients' continuity of care; cooperation between the two programs produces seamless care for patients and their families.

For example, we saw a young man with progressive lung disease who had had multiple septic episodes and was on a ventilator. After several months in this condition, his last request was to see his home one final time and then to return to the ICU to have the ventilator withdrawn. With the hospice's help, we arranged for the patient to be taken home by ambulance. The hospice's health care providers who were experienced with ventilator management, accompanied him. Then he returned to the hospital and died soon after removal of the ventilator.

In the first year, we built a number of links to the UPMC Hospice. Its director, Carol DeMoss, R.N., M.S.N., serves on the Palliative Care Service Steering Committee and attends all weekly multidisciplinary meetings. David Pasquale, D.O. (doctor of osteopathy), a consulting physician, was medical co-director of the hospice with Dr. Linda King. (When Dr. Pasquale left palliative care in January 2000, Dr. King became the sole medical director.)

In addition to coordinating their clinical efforts, the Palliative Care Service and UPMC Hospice have cooperated on administration and fund-raising. We jointly raised more than $102,000 in 1999 through cookbook sales, theater parties, and general solicitations. The largest portion of funds was raised by the Development Center,

which sponsored a children's ball that raised over $50,000. We have also worked together to develop clinical guidelines on treating delirium and have held joint educational programs for the hospice staff.

Pittsburgh has more than 20 other hospices. We hope to build relationships with them in the upcoming years to improve palliative care. Our first project will be to agree on ways to measure nausea and to set standards for its treatment.

We also plan to expand our efforts to stress palliative care for social workers and nurses. One of the social workers who has been most active in palliative care is developing a curriculum for social work students to increase their exposure to palliative care and hospice. We are developing educational sessions for social workers at UPMC-Presbyterian and UPMC-Shadyside. The palliative care nurse practitioner is developing a curriculum for oncology nurse practitioners. He is also preparing a monthlong rotation in palliative care for nursing students and nurse practitioner students. We will continue working with nurses on the medical and surgical units to improve their ability to provide palliative care.

We also plan to expand our bereavement program. In the next year we want to:

- develop a similar program at UPMC-Shadyside;

- create a monthly bereavement support group; and
- develop a more effective way to screen people at high risk of complicated grief.

Regarding this last item, investigators at Western Psychiatric Institute and Clinic have developed a highly reliable screening tool for "traumatic grief." This tool has not been widely used in non-research settings. We would like to work with these researchers to identify family members who need intensive interventions to decrease their psychiatric morbidity.

Since the spring of 1999, a number of new opportunities have developed for the Palliative Care Service: (1) The anesthesia-based Chronic Pain Service has stopped doing inpatient consultation, allowing the Service to expand its non-terminal pain care. (2) The University of Pittsburgh Cancer Institute has funding to obtain cancer tissues from recently deceased patients; the tissue will then be studied molecularly and short- and long-term cell cultures will be developed. Our Service will see outpatients with terminal prostate, colon, and breast cancer and help obtain their consent for this study. We will therefore have an opportunity to see that palliative care is available to these patients. (3) We have been asked to develop a two-week curriculum for all critical care medicine fellows. (4) The University of Pittsburgh received a Geriatric Research and Evaluation Clinical Center (GRECC) focusing on strokes. This opens new opportunities for collaborative research on advance directives and end-of-life care. (5) Investigators at Western Psychiatric Institute and Clinic have recently been funded to study traumatic grief. They have asked us to help them enroll hospice patients. (6) Frequent admissions from nursing homes to certain UPMC Health Care System hospitals has led to discussion of whether palliative care consultations can decrease this repetitive process. The lesson is that the Service needs to remain flexible and alert to opportunities that arise within the University of Pittsburgh Health Care System. (7) The Institute for Performance Improvement hired a social worker to provide psychosocial support for families of critically ill patients. This social worker has extensive palliative care experience and has become an invaluable part of our team.

Looking Back

Building the Comprehensive Palliative Care Service has, in large part, been a very positive experience. Our significant accomplishments include designing and developing the Service, gaining acceptance within the hospitals, obtaining feedback from families who report that we really helped them, and developing educational programs to teach others how to provide better palliative care. While our success has been gratifying, we have had growing pains. If we could start anew, I would probably do three things differently.

First, I would have discussed the goals of palliative care with other physicians in greater detail and would have done a better job of negotiating how we could meet these goals. I envisaged the Service as a 24-hour-a-day, seven-day-a-week program to help doctors take better care of terminally ill patients. I do not want to limit the program only to patients who have accepted death or who simply want comfort care; this goal was not shared by the other physicians. Second, I would have done a better job of communicating with social workers and making them a central part of the Service. Third, I would have built a better decision-making structure. Too much of the program was tied to me. In a hurry to get going, I made unilateral decisions that should have been made by a palliative care committee. This is not a healthy administrative structure and keeps other participants from feeling valued and limits their contributions. To counteract this, we now hold quarterly retreats at which we discuss our program and its progress and direction. The recent addition of a senior faculty member in palliative care who is eager to share administrative responsibilities

has been helpful.

I am not sure how to guarantee the survival of the Comprehensive Palliative Care Service. We cannot sustain ourselves as a clinical entity, because our clinical income will not support the multidisciplinary team. My immediate goal is to promote our research activities. In an academic institution, long-term viability is tied to one's ability to do research and obtain research money. We have begun to develop a group of colleagues interested in palliative care research. We have submitted a number of grant proposals and will continue to seek research funding.

PAID STAFF

Robert Arnold, MD*	Director Palliative Care Service	25% support for administering program + 4 months on service
Linda King, MD*	Director of UPMC Hospice	10% for hospice activities + 5 months on service
Paul Han, MD, MA*	Attending physician	3 months
David Pasquale, DO#*	Attending physician	3 months
Michael Devita, MD	Attending physician	1 month
Raymond Paronish, CRNP*	Nurse practitioner	100%
Lyda Dye, RN, MSN	Administrative director	10%
Mary Ellen Cowan, MSW	Administrative support	5%
Lisa Painter, RN	Administrative support	5%
To be hired	Secretary	50%

VOLUNTEER STAFF

Rowena Schwartz, PharmD	Pain consultant
Ellen Redinbaugh, PhD	Psychologist
Father Sam Esposito	Clerical consultant
Joyce Herschl, MSW	Clinical social worker
Carol DeMoss, RN, MSN	Manager, UPMC Home Hospice
Ione Miller	UPCI
Lisa Hartley	Volunteer coordinator
David Barnard, PhD	Educational program director
Beth Chaitin, MSW, MA	Clinical social worker
Carolyn Longest	Volunteer
Barbara Dippold	Volunteer
Nicole Fowler	Volunteer

* Supported by clinical revenue

April 1998–June 1999

A. Name of program: UPMC Comprehensive Palliative Care Service

B. Program director: Robert Arnold, MD

C. Program start-date: 1996

D. Institutional setting: Urban

E. Type of institution: Academic; affiliated medical school: University of Pittsburgh Schools of Health Sciences

F. Number of beds: 1,295 (Presbyterian University Hospital has 809 licensed beds; Shadyside University Hospital has 486 licensed beds.)

G. Health care system:

    1. Number of hospital affiliates in health care system: 24

    2. Number of long-term care affiliates in health care system:

        a. 9 skilled nursing units in hospitals

        b. 10 freestanding facilities offering independent living, assisted living, and skilled nursing options

TOTAL PATIENTS FROM APRIL 1998 TO NOVEMBER 1999: 694

Age: 62 Avg (17 yrs. to 100 yrs.)

Ethnicity

White	79%
Black	19%
Hispanic	1%
Asian	1%

Site of Discharge

Died at discharge	35%
Hospice	27%
Inpatient Hospice	3%
Home Care	3%
Nursing Home	13%
Other:	19%

Sex

Male	52%
Female	48%

Diagnosis

Cancer	58%
Stroke/Coma	12%
End-Stage Heart Disease	7%
End-Stage Lung Disease	7%
End-Stage Liver Disease	5%
End-Stage Renal Disease	3%
HIV	2%
Other	6%

Revenues $67,988

Sources of Revenues*

Medicare	64%
Commercial	11% (including self-paying patients)
PA Medical Assistance	10%
Managed Care Medical Assistance	5%
PA Blue Shield	7%
Keystone (HMO/POS)	5%

*Total exceeds 100% due to rounding.

University of Pittsburgh Medical Center Hospitals
Comprehensive Palliative Care Service
Funding Sources, July–December 1999*

Medicare	62%	
Commercial (including private party)	11%	
PA Medical Assistance	10%	
PA Blue Shield	7%	
Managed Care Medical Assistance	5%	
Keystone (HMO/POS)	5%	

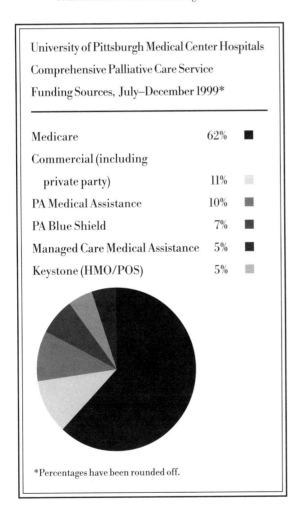

*Percentages have been rounded off.

ACTIVE

PI (primary investigator): Arnold	01/01/99–06/30/00	15% (donated)
The Greenwall Foundation	$92,736	

Evaluating the Impact of Financial Incentives on Organ Donation

The investigative team will use past research and adopt existing tools to evaluate the impact of incentives on the attitudes and willingness of families to consent to organ donation requests.

Co-PI: Arnold	11/01/98–10/31/00	10% (donated)
Nathan Cummings Foundation	$80,500	

Physicians' Reactions to Patients' Deaths

The impetus for this study is based on observations that physicians' emotions play a significant role in the way they deal with dying patients.

PI: Roberts	07/01/97–06/30/00	2.5% (donated)
HRSA	$190,000	

Faculty Development in GIM and/or GP

This grant is meant to provide further training for physicians in patient care, teaching, research, and administration.

PI: Degenholtz	04/01/99–03/31/00	2.5%
Subcontract: Univ of Massachusetts	$70,441	

Informed Consent Research

Therapeutic misconception involves patients/subjects failing to grasp the difference between participating in clinical research and receiving ordinary clinical care.

PI: Tabas	07/01/99–06/30/00	10%
HRSA	$270,000	

General Internal Medicine and General Internal Pediatrics Residency Training

This project is meant to complete the conversion of the Shadyside Hospital Internal Medicine Residency Program from a traditional program to a General Internal Medicine Residency, with an emphasis on primary care.

Co-Investigator: Arnold   08/01/99–07/31/00   10%

Co-Investigator: Redinbaugh   30%

NIH $100,000

An Intervention to Improve End-of-Life Family Care

The study tests the efficacy of a stress and coping intervention for cancer patients and their family caregivers.

PI: Arnold   07/01/97–06/30/02   60%

Open Society Institute $70,000

Teaching Physician Change-Agents to Communicate with Terminally Ill Patients about Psychosocial and Ethical Aspects of Care

The goal of this project is to develop, implement, and evaluate a model for improving practicing physicians' communication with terminally ill patients regarding psychological and ethical aspects of their care.

PI: Redinbaugh   08/01/99–07/31/00   20%

Consultant: Arnold

National Institute on Aging $50,000

Improving the quality of life at the end of life.

This project tests the effectiveness of educating family caregivers about managing pain and loss of appetite at the very end of life.

PI: Paronish   1999–2000   5%

Co-PI: Arnold   2% (donated)

Beckwith Foundation $3,500

Developing a Palliative Care Unit: Promoting Nurse Competencies

This project involves the creation and use of a structured curriculum to improve nurses' knowledge of and attitudes toward palliative care.

PI: Arnold   01/01/00–12/31/00   NA

Ladies Hospital Aid Society $5,000

Support for the UPMC Palliative Care Program

This grant provides support for the inpatient palliative care program and the bereavement
program.

PENDING

PI: Barnard   05/01/00–04/30/01   NA

University of Pittsburgh

Provost's Innovation in Education Award Program

Learning from Patients with Life-Threatening Illness

This project involves the development of a curriculum to improve first-year students' knowledge
of and attitudes toward caring for individuals with life-limiting illnesses.

PI: Degenholtz   07/01/00–06/30/03

Co-Investigator: Arnold   5%

AHCPR

The Effect of Nursing Home Residents' Advance Directives

This study will examine the effect of advance directives on the care of nursing home residents
and the cost of care.

PI: Chelluri   07/01/00–03/31/03

Co-PI: Arnold   10%

NIH $1,068,006

Intensive Support for Families During Critical Illness

We propose regular meetings between families and clinicians to discuss patients' medical
condition and prognosis, patient/family views and preferences about life-sustaining treatment.

PI: Bryce   07/01/00–06/30/05

Co-PI: Arnold   5%

NIH $470,221

Estimating ESLD Prevalence and Treatment Variation

This project evaluates the role of gender, race, and income in determining access to liver

transplantation and explaining variation in liver transplant rates.

PI: Roberts   07/01/00–06/30/03

Co-Investigator: Arnold   2.5%

HRSA $1,274,239

Faculty Development in General Internal Medicine

This grant is meant to provide more training for physicians in patient care, teaching, research,

and administration.

PI: Degenholtz

Co-Investigator: Arnold   5%

NIH/NIA $50,000

Prevalence and Use of Advance Directives among the Oldest Old

The proposed study will use data from proxy informants for sample members who died before

their 1995 follow-up interview.

PI: Siminoff   12/01/00–11/30/05

Co-PI: Arnold   20%

Subcontract: Case Western Reserve Univ. $147,379

Increasing Consent to Organ Donation: A Randomized Trial

This study is meant to increase the number of organs donated for transplants.

PI: Barnard   04/01/01–03/31/05

Co-PI: Arnold

National Cancer Institute $697,892

Undergraduate Medical Education for End of Life Care

The goal of this project is a four-year medical school curriculum in which each year makes the optimal,

stage-appropriate contribution to effective and compassionate care of patients near the end of life.

A complete list of the Fund's reports may be viewed online at www.milbank.org. Copies of print editions of reports are available without charge. Most reports are also available electronically on the Fund's Web site.

The Education of Medical Students: Ten Stories of Curriculum Change
co-published with the Association of American Medical Colleges
2000   248 pages

Long-Term Care for the Elderly with Disabilities: Current Policy, Emerging Trends, and Implications for the Twenty-First Century
by Robyn I. Stone
2000   96 pages

Better Information, Better Outcomes? The Use of Health Technology Assessment and Clinical Effectiveness Data in Health Care Purchasing Decisions in the United Kingdom and the United States
2000   36 pages

Genetics in Medicine: Real Promises, Unreal Expectations. One Scientist's Advice to Policymakers in the United Kingdom and the United States
by Steve Jones
2000   28 pages

Effective Public Management of Mental Health Care: Views from States on Medicaid Reforms that Enhance Service Integration and Accountability
co-published with the Bazelon Center for Mental Health Law
2000   56 pages

Principles for Care of Patients at the End of Life: An Emerging Consensus among the Specialties of Medicine
by Christine K. Cassel and Kathleen M. Foley
1999   32 pages

Patients as Effective Collaborators in Managing Chronic Conditions
co-published with the Center for the Advancement of Health
1999   32 pages

New Foundations in Health: Six Stories
1999   168 pages

End-of-Life Care and Hospital Legal Counsel: Current Involvement and Opportunities for the Future
by Connie Zuckerman with an introduction by Robert A. Burt and Christine K. Cassel
co-published with the United Hospital Fund
1999   44 pages

Public-Private Collaboration in Health Information Policy
co-published with the Reforming States Group
1999   32 pages

1997 State Health Care Expenditure Report
co-published with the National Association of State Budget Officers and the Reforming States Group
1999   192 pages

Enhancing the Accountability of Alternative Medicine
1998   44 pages

Improving State Law to Prevent and Treat Infectious Disease
by Lawrence O. Gostin, Scott Burris, Zita Lazzarini, and Kathleen Maguire
1998   56 pages

The following books are available from their publishers, Aspen Publishers (1-800-638-8437); Blackwell Publishers (1-800-216-2522); Oxford University Press (1-800-451-7556); and University of California Press (1-800-822-6657).

THE CALIFORNIA/MILBANK SERIES ON HEALTH AND THE PUBLIC
co-published with and distributed by the University of California Press

Public Health Law: Power, Duty, Restraint
by Lawrence O. Gostin
California/Milbank Series, 3
Available January 2001   518 pages
$60.00 cloth; $24.95 paper

Experiencing Politics: A Legislator's Stories of Government and Health Care
by John E. McDonough
California/Milbank Series, 2
Available November 2000   336 pages
$50.00 cloth; $19.95 paper

The Corporate Practice of Medicine: Competition and Innovation in Physician Organization
by James C. Robinson
California/Milbank Series, 1
1999   306 pages
$45.00 cloth; $18.95 paper

OTHER BOOKS

Doctoring: The Nature of Primary Care Medicine
by Eric J. Cassell
1997   224 pages
co-published with and distributed by
Oxford University Press $27.50

Treating Drug Abusers Effectively
edited by Daniel M. Fox, Joel A. Egertson, and Alan I. Leshner
1997   368 pages
co-published with and distributed by
Blackwell Publishers $62.95

Home-Based Care for a New Century
edited by Daniel M. Fox and Carol Raphael
1997   320 pages
co-published with and distributed by
Blackwell Publishers $70.95

Public Health Leaders Tell Their Stories
edited by Lloyd F. Novick, Carol Spain Woltring, and Daniel M. Fox
1997   192 pages
co-published with and distributed by Aspen Publishers $38.00

The Fund also publishes the *Milbank Quarterly*, a journal of public health and health care policy. Information about subscribing to the *Quarterly* is available by calling toll-free 1-800-835-6770, or at www.milbank.org/quarterly/

Information about other work of the Fund is available from the Fund at 645 Madison Ave., 15th Floor, New York, NY 10022, (212)355-8400. Fax: (212)355-8599. E-mail: mmf@milbank.org. On the Web: www.milbank.org

*Precepts of Palliative Care**
1997   4 pages (for professionals)
*A Vision for Better Care at the End of Life**
1998   2 pages (for lay audiences)
Last Acts Task Force on Palliative Care
Available through Stewart Communications,
312-642-8652

*State Initiatives in End-of-Life Care: Policy
Guide for State Legislators**
Dick Merritt, Wendy Fox-Grage, et al.
June 1998   48 pages

*Advances in State Pain Policy and
Medical Practice**
In the series State Initiatives in End-of-Life
Care, issue 4
April 1999   8 pages

*The Challenge of End-of-Life Care: Moving
Toward Metanoia?**
Last Acts Financing Task Force
October 1998   22 pages

"Unexpected Returns: Insights from
SUPPORT"
by Joanne Lynn
In *To Improve Health and Health Care
1998: The Robert Wood Johnson Foundation
Anthology*, eds. S.L. Isaacs and J.R.
Knickman, 161–86
San Francisco: Jossey-Bass Publishers, 1997

The SUPPORT Project to Improve Care at
the End of Life (video)
by Ben Achtenberg
Boston: Fanlight Productions
Available through Fanlight Productions,
(800) 937-4113
or on the Web: www.fanlight.com

For information on placing an order (except as noted above), call the Communications
Department of the Robert Wood Johnson Foundation: (609) 951-5753. Asterisked items are
available on the Last Acts Web site: www.lastacts.org. Click on "Precepts of Palliative Care" for
the first item and "Publications" for the others.

Copyeditor:

Marie Shear

Design and Typography:

Watts Design? Inc.

Printing:

Prestone Printing Company, Inc.